HANDBOOK OF
CENTRAL AUDITORY PROCESSING
DISORDERS IN CHILDREN

HANDBOOK OF CENTRAL AUDITORY PROCESSING DISORDERS IN CHILDREN

Jack A. Willeford, Ph.D.

Professor of Audiology
Colorado State University
Director, Royal Arch Research Assistance
Program of Central Auditory Processing Disorders
Fort Collins, Colorado

Joan M. (Billger) Burleigh, M.A.

Instructor of Audiology
Colorado State University
Assistant Director, Royal Arch Research Assistance
Program of Central Auditory Processing Disorders
Fort Collins, Colorado

Grune & Stratton, Inc.
(Harcourt Brace Jovanovich, Publishers)
Orlando   San Diego   New York
London   Toronto   Montreal   Sydney   Tokyo

Library of Congress Cataloging-in-Publication Data

Willeford, Jack A.
  Handbook of central auditory processing disorders in children.
  Bibliography: p.
  1. Hearing disorders in children—Complications
and sequelae. 2. Speech disorders in children.
3. Language disorders in children. 4. Learning
disabilities. 5. Auditory perception in children.
6. Perception, Disorders of. I. Burleigh, Joan M.
II. Title. [DNLM: 1. Perceptual Disorders—in
infancy & childhood. WV 272 W698h]
RF291.5.C45W53 1985   618.92′855   85-10084
ISBN 0-8089-1727-7

Grune & Stratton, Inc.
Orlando, FL 32887

Distributed in the United Kingdom by
Grune & Stratton, Ltd.
24/28 Oval Road, London NW 1

Library of Congress Catalog Number 85-10084
International Standard Book Number 0-8089-1727-7
Printed in the United States of America
85 86 87 88   10 9 8 7 6 5 4 3 2 1

Contents

Acknowledgments

We extend our deepest gratitude to the Royal Arch Masons, International, whose support has helped to make possible many of the efforts discussed in this book. This assistance has been made possible by the creation of the Royal Arch Research Assistance Foundation. Our thanks go to Ms. Liz Lambert for her skilled typing of the text, and to Bruce Pierce, Ph.D., for his helpful technical assistance. Special appreciation is extended to Andrew J. Burleigh, M.S., for his insightful editorial critique of the manuscript. Finally, we wish to thank our families for their support and patience during the writing of this book.

Preface

This book presents the essence of approximately twelve years of experience by the authors in dealing with children having central auditory processing disorders (CAPD).* Our purpose is to share the knowledge gained through this experience in the hope that it may have value for other professionals, the parents of such children, and, in the final analysis, the children themselves. Much of the material is original information, but we have also drawn on the contributions of others. Many of the concepts and practices that are presented have developed from our own experiences in working with children with deficiencies of the central auditory nervous system (CANS). Our discussion will include the difficulties inherent in defining CAPD, theories concerning the causes of such problems, the behaviors manifested by children with CAPD, associated social, academic, and language problems, diagnostic methods, and treatment strategies.

The subject matter is somewhat controversial, as will become apparent. This is partly due, we believe, to the diverse philosophies concerning this disorder. Current understanding is impeded by virtue of the fact that we are still unraveling the complexities of the CANS itself. Moreover, acoustic signals are highly transitory when compared with visual stimuli whether the latter be pictures, numbers, or written language. Visual stimuli can be held motionless and critically analyzed in every detail; they can be viewed from various distances and angles, in different shades of lighting, or with varying degrees of magnification; they can be isolated relatively easily from other competing or intruding visual stimuli; and, finally, they can be viewed, in many instances, for as long as one desires. Impressive scientific advancements have also been made in computer-assisted techniques for enhancing figure-ground clarity of visual objects in our space programs, in meteorological science, and in military map reading of aerial photographs.

Advances in acoustic technology have not been as rapid, partciularly when applied to verbal signals. In addition to lacking the advantage of our being able to suspend them in the dimension of time, typical acoustic signals are in constant stages of change. Their characteristics are modified

---

*The use of acronyms in this text will be limited to those which are commonly used and only in those contexts where their use facilitates the ease of reading.

by numerous variables. Speech, in particular, is altered by factors such as fundamental frequency, intensity, speed, articulation, voice inflection, emotional emphasis, distance from the source, and the countless juxtapositions of words and their phonemic and subphonemic elements in continuous discourse. Finally, auditory signals for the purpose of human communication are often received in the presence of dynamically changing competition from a host of other auditory signals pervading our daily-living environments. Thus, it seems truly miraculous that humans are endowed with auditory capabilities that permit them to sort out desired signals from complex auditory environments and process them through an elaborate series of delicately balanced CANS mechanisms. These mechanisms transmit, enhance or inhibit, reshape, refine, and/or modify them in numerous ways and ultimately assign recognition and meaning to them. The end result allows us to respond with meaningful behaviors, most especially to communicate thoughts and ideas, to learn and develop intellectually and emotionally. Most people can and do perform this phenomenal task with relative ease in an often complex and bewildering world in which our sensory systems are bombarded with myriad signals. This fact inspires appreciation for the intricately dsigned sensory and neural systems which human beings enjoy. However, all of the foregoing factors conspire, at times, to deceive and confuse even the normal listener, as we all know. Consider, then, how different (indeed, how difficult) life must be for the individual with imperfections in that processing machinery. Through a variety of physical, mental, emotional, or maturational limitations, regardless of cause, many people are unable to make efficient use of the sensory information they receive from their environments. One such population is comprised of those children with central auditory deficiencies that lead to communication difficulties and their attendant academic and social impacts. It is these children and their families to whom this book is dedicated, in order that we might make their role in the auditory world a better one, and one with a brighter future.

Introduction

Children with central auditory disorders present unique problems for their parents, their teachers, and for the many professionals who are called upon to evaluate and prescribe management for a given child's communication problems and resulting academic and social difficulties. Such children, by the fundamental nature of their disorder, pose a special challenge for audiologists and speech-language pathologists, as well as for other specialists and classroom teachers. They do so because they present with a *communication disorder* in the broadest sense of the term, a disorder that encompasses considerably more than a specific language disorder. These are chidren who have difficulty in correctly perceiving spoken language and other meaningful sounds in their environments. This difficulty may be due, in some children, to a deficiency in basic linguistic capabilities, but in others it may be due to faulty auditory perception that has no apparent relationship to the child's language skills. Both types of children exhibit these problems in spite of the fact that they are found to have peripheral auditory systems that operate absolutely normally in response to basic and traditional measures of auditory functions. For example, children with central auditory disorders demonstrate excellent sensitivity on pure tone tests, except for a mild-to-moderate impairment at 8000 Hz in an undetermined but substantial number of them (Pinheiro, 1977b; Willeford, 1980a). They also typically have normal speech reception thresholds, and they score within normal limits on standardized audiological tests of speech discrimination ability. Thus, such children readily pass the pure tone screening examinations administered when referred by teachers to rule out the existence of a possible loss of hearing. Yet, they have difficulty in understanding or utilizing auditory information on their academic and social environments and present case histories describing behaviors that, indeed, support the suspicions of teachers, parents, and peers that they do not use auditory information efficiently. However, the processes involved in eliciting a response to pure tones—or in accurately repeating highly-controlled, redundant, and easily audible verbal stimuli of the type used in traditional speech audiometry—is not always a formidable task, a fact for which we establish a neurophysiological base in Chapter 2. Such tests are routinely administered in an audiological test suite in which the control of both the listening environment and the test signals is optimized. This is a markedly different task from that of receiving and integrating the complex and dynamically changing auditory signals present in the classroom, on the playground, or in home and community environments. These are the situations in which the child with a *central auditory processing disorder* (CAPD) fails to perform as expected whether it be in academic achievement or in social conduct. Such a lack of normal performance arouses concern in parents and teachers and leads to frustration, anxiety, and bewilderment in the child. His* practical use of the auditory stimuli in his daily living environment is limited because he appears to have a *central auditory nervous system* (CANS) that inefficiently sorts out and process the meaningful auditory signals in his world. This problem is not easily recognized by professionals in many areas, particularly communication disorders, education, psychology, and pediatrics. This is due, in the authors' judgment, to the following reasons:

1. Knowledge of CANS anatomy and physiology is still extremely limited.
2. Traditional auditory tests are not designed to assess complex CANS processes, especially in individuals with subtle disorders.
3. Professional judgments are too frequently based on theories that are not adequately confirmed by reality, particularly in terms of auditory-linguistic relationships.
4. Such disorders are viewed too simplistically.
5. Terminology is often vague and inappropriate.
6. Meaningful interdisciplinary dialogue about such problems has been extremely limited.

Professional activity in the area of communication disorders serves as an ideal illustration. In spite of the common coursework in our undergraduate training programs, and in spite of our common interests in persons with communication disorders, our graduate education models in audiology and speech-language pathology and our individual interests lead us to isolated areas of expertise. This is evident from the nature of the activities we pursue in our studies and from the diverse clinical endeavors we pursue as they relate to individuals with CANS disorders. The result

---

*Use of the pronoun *he* is used in this text to facilitate discussion, and because of the substantially greater number of boys reported to have such disorders.

is that we have two groups of specialists in communication disorders working independently on a problem that often has common features, but doing so with diverse philosophies, using dissimilar diagnostic instruments, and employing intervention strategies that are generally quite different. It is the author's present position that while we are making progress, neither group sufficiently understands the nature of the problem. This conclusion is based on the fact that, as the number of such children seen professionally increases, the greater the insights develop that fail to support some of the theories that we previously held sacred. Such is the caution that Rees (1973) advised in her article, "Auditory Processing Factors in Language Disorders: The View from Procrustes' Bed." Perhaps we too often complicate the problems we attempt to resolve by combining our present concepts of central auditory processing disorders with those of language disorders as though they involved a simple cause-and-effect relationship. The latter are also in need of much further definition and resolution. That should not be surprising, since language disorders involve the myriad intricacies of speaking, listening, reading, and writing. These intricacies are further confounded by the complexities involved in *learning disabilities* (LD). We complicate the problems in search for, and solutions to, difficulties experienced by children who fail to perform academically and socially in ways that are predicted for them by traditional yardsticks of measurement. The following sections explore these factors in greater detail.

LEARNING DISABILITIES

The area of LD has intrigued professionals for many generations. Physicians have investigated the etiologies of LD since the beginning of the nineteenth century, according to Wiederholt (1978). One of the first and best-known physicians involved in the study of LD was Franz Joseph Gall, who worked with brain-injured adults (Gearheart, 1981). Other physicians followed suit, and the majority of work centered on the categorization of different types of LD in adults with acquired brain injuries (Wiederholt, 1978). Many of these adults were aphasic, and physicians tried to localize the area of damage in the brain.

Eventually, information regarding brain-injured children and their learning capabilities began to accumulate. Even as early as the 1860s and 1870s investigators questioned whether or not children who sustained a brain injury that resulted in a mental deficiency should be classified differently from those children who evidenced lower intellectual capacity of primarily genetic origin (Gearheart, 1977).

Although many individuals were already involved in studying brain dysfunction and its effect on mental capabilities, learning disabilities was not truly established as an inclusive field of study until Strauss and Lehtinen (1947) published their widely acclaimed *Psychopathology and Education of the Brain-injured Child*. After working with brain-injured veterans in Germany, Strauss shifted his attention to U.S. school-aged children who were experiencing academic difficulties. Many of the children with whom Strauss worked had language and visual-motor difficulties and often demonstrated hyperkinetic tendencies. Many of these chiildren also seemed to perform well in certain academic areas while performing at a very low level in others.

Interest in LD has progressed steadily since those bold pioneering efforts, and many other individuals have made important contributions to this emerging discipline. Some of the more notable included Samuel Orton, Heinz Werner, Helmer Myklebust, Newell Kephart, Marianne Frostig, and William Cruickshank, all of whom are recognized for their work in various aspects of the area of LD. Their investigations span avenues of perceptual-motor disabilities, figure-ground disturbances, hyperkinesia, visual-perceptual disorders, language-learning disabilities, and auditory perceptual deficiencies. Through their efforts, and the accumulated research of others, a considerable body of knowledge has developed to aid children who are working below their academic potential. This experience culminated in the enactment of PL 94-142 (1975) amended as follows, which defines children with specific learning disabilities:

"Specific learning disability" means a disorder in one or more of the basic psychological processes involved in understanding or in using language, spoken or written, which may manifest itself in an imperfect ability to listen, think, speak, read, write, spell, or to do mathematical calculations. The term includes such conditions as perceptual handicaps, brain injury, minimal brain dysfunction, dyslexia, and developmental aphasia. The term does not include children who have learning problems which are primarily the result of visual, hearing, or motor handicaps, of mental retardation, of emotional disturbance, or environmental, cultural, or economic disadvantage (Section 121(a)(5), 1977).

The National Joint Committee of Learning Disabilities (NJCLD) is a group of professionals representing the American Speech-Language-Hearing Association, the Association for Children and Adults with Learning Disabilities, the Council for Learning Disabilities, the Division of Children with Communication Disorders, the International Reading Association, and the Orton Dyslexia Society. This group adopted a revised definition of LD in 1981 that reads as follows:

Learning disabilities is a generic term that refers to a heterogeneous group of disorders manifested by significant difficulties in the acquisition and use of listening, speaking, reading, writing, reasoning, or mathematical abilities. These disorders are intrinsic to the individual and presumed to be due to central nervous system dysfunction. Even though a learning disability may occur concomitantly with other handicapping conditions (e.g., sensory impairment, mental retardation, social and emotional disturbance) or environmental influences (e.g., cultural differences, insufficient/inappropriate instruction, psychogenic factors), it is not the direct result of those conditions or influences (Hammill, Leigh, McNutt, & Larson, 1981).

This latest definition suggests a swing to placing greater emphasis on central nervous system dysfunction. Such a focus has also been embraced by the Canadian ACLD, which defines LD as "a heterogeneous group of disorders due to identifiable or inferred central nervous system damage" (Moser, 1983).

Auditory and language factors, in particular, have captured the imagination of many professionals, especially those in speech-language pathology and audiology. While this interest has led to the advancement of our knowledge, it has also muddied the scientific and clinical waters. Perhaps the latter is the result of drawing too heavily on remote, often dated literature, some of which may be more analogous than relevant. Unfortunately, theories, tests, and treatment programs have been developed that are based on such literature.

THE AUDITORY PROCESSING OF LANGUAGE

That audition plays a fundamental role in the development and use of language is self-evident. Ample support for such a relationship may be found in the vastly diverse languages that are spoken among people of different ethnic groups around the earth, in the dialectical differences within single ethnic groups, in the profound influence on language resulting from deafness in young children, and even in the impact of simple deprivation in children with normal hearing (Curtiss, 1977). The danger (and perhaps the only danger) in immediate acceptance of such convincing evidence lies in the degree to which it is generalized for teaching or clinical purposes. Impressive research has advanced our knowledge substantially with regard to the perception of certain sub-elements of spoken language and has led to the formulation of theoretical models that appear to have been interpreted too liberally by many clinicians.

A common feature of several theoretical models proposes that auditory perceptual processes involve a hierarchy of operational levels that range from an initial acoustic analysis, through stages of phonetic, phonological, and syntactic analyses, to the ultimate levels of semantic analysis. An excellent review of this literature by Levy (1981) suggests that these models follow from carefully designed and executed studies of vowel and consonant recognition, the most valuable of which have been conducted with synthetic speech. The synthetic stimulus permits greater control of, or reduces the variances in, the acoustic signals studied; it also permits systematic modifications of the signals under study. The works of Hirsh (1967), Stevens and House (1972), Studdert-Kennedy (1974), and Pisoni and Sawusch (1975) are among several noteworthy studies of language-element processing in normal subjects.

In most theoretical models, the speech signal is initially analyzed in a manner that permits the sorting, coding, and transmission of intensity, frequency, and temporal characteristics to the next level where distinctive phonetic feature analyses are conducted. The latter product is then transformed into the higher-level operations of syntactical, cognitive, and semantic processing. Unfortunately, such theories are difficult to substantiate because consonant-vowel combinations (CVs), the signals of choice since they are easier to manage acoustically than expanded language segments, are abstractions of speech and thus difficult to translate to the elusive nature of the complex auditory signals that comprise conversational speech. Moreover, Liberman, Copper, Shankweiler, and Studdert-Kennedy (1967) have shown that, even with the assistance of synthetically-generated speech signals of highly restricted content, there is some lack of correspondence between units of acoustic signals and those of lingusitic analysis. Such a result confirms that the precise nature of how acoustic signals trigger linguistic events is still beyond our understanding. It would be most helpful if one could look inside the human head with some precision instrument and visualize these processes as they occur. Block (1983) has argued convincingly that mental pictures are an important part of cognition, but their neurophysiologic bases are equally mystifying to scientists. Perhaps we will never really know how these phenomena function, although recent scientific advances in mapping neurological images of electrical activity in the stimulated central auditory nervous system show promise (Duffy, Burchfiel, & Lambroso, 1980). Still another method involves the use of magnetoencephalograms (MEG) for defining neurological function (Reite, Zimmerman, & Zimmerman, 1981). Unfortunately, as they involve auditory studies, these techniques presently employ single, repetitive signals, and it may be years before the intricate processes of complex speech perception yield to resolution. It would seem prudent to search for further neurophysiologic bases for what truly is one of life's great miracles. For the present, however, it is feasible to accomplish this clinical task with the classical stimulus-response paradigm using phonemes, words, and sentences as stimuli.

PHILOSOPHIES OF EVALUATING
CENTRAL AUDITORY FUNCTION

Speech-Language Approach

Knowledge of the existing research, and our need to appreciate the clinical implications of communication deficiencies in certain children, have provided the major impetus for the development of most contemporary approaches to the measurement of central auditory function. Other approaches have sprung from efforts to factor out a variety of perceptual subskills that are presumed by some authorities to be essential elements of the phonemenon (or phenomena) often referred to as "auditory processing" or "auditory perception" (Aten, 1972; Butler, 1975; Flowers, Costello & Small, 1970; Kirk, McCarthy, & Kirk, 1968; Rampp, 1980; Wiig & Semel, 1976; Witkin, 1971; Wood, 1972). Some of the more commonly labeled components used by these authors, and others, include but are not limited to the following theoretical skills. The reader is urged to think about what they mean independent of definitions in the literature.

1. Auditory analysis
2. Auditory closure
3. Auditory discrimination
4. Auditory comprehension
5. Auditory association
6. Auditory attention
7. Auditory memory (short term)
8. Auditory memory (long term)
9. Auditory sequencing
10. Auditory synthesis
11. Auditory vigilance.

Terms such as these are generally defended on the basis of a given theoretical model, and/or are descriptive of certain covert neurophysiologic activities that are presumed to occur in the communication process. Unfortunately, the same terms are used differently by different authors (Butler, 1980; Willeford & Billger, 1978).[†] Apparently this is the result of differences in either definition or interpretation, or perhaps an effort to

---

[†]The following definitions serve as an example. Butler (1980) refers to auditory attention as sensory processes that increase the probability of detecting anticipated auditory events, whereas Rampp (1980) defines it as the ability to focus selectively for increased lengths of time on a task or series of tasks.

improve on the original concept. The problem is not in the labeling process itself, but in the use of such labels to constitute some sort of truths about real neurophysiologic events.

Many tests have been developed that purport to isolate and evaluate important subelements, listed earlier, of central auditory events that are necessary for language processes to occur. Descriptions in test manuals and/or in associated literature include references to measurement of such factors, or are used by writers to describe elements of auditory behavior that are presumed to facilitate the understanding of verbal signals (Aten, 1972; Barr, 1972; Butler, 1980; Flowers et al, 1970; Kirk et al, 1968; Rampp, 1980; Witkin, 1971; Wood, 1972). These "auditory" descriptors are used to explain or describe specific events that are believed to take place in the process of receiving and understanding verbal stimuli such that language processes are set in motion. They stem largely from theoretical models that are assumed to be important aspects of real processes. More often than not, however, they are based on theoretical principles of language development and language use and are impossible to isolate independently and define in clinical assessment, since, as acknowledged by Witkin (1971), many of these concepts appear to overlap or to occur in complicated simultaneous relationships, so that it is difficult to determine which concept is being evaluated. The Auditory Perception Training (APT) training tapes [‡] are an illustration of this problem. These tapes were designed to train diverse aspects of audition, yet many involve tasks that are quite similar and overlap with requirements on other tapes that are supposed to train different auditory skills. Nonetheless, it is not uncommon for researchers to develop a single-feature test with little or no attempt to relate it to more global processes. In our view, we simply do not know how to isolate or measure these circumscribed functions. At present, the degree to which any of them are important in themselves or in combination with other factors in some critical anatomical, temporal, or acoustical relationship is largely unknown. Despite the uncertainties, some interesting postulations about auditory perceptual processes have been developed (Weener, 1974).

Even though numerous tests have been developed that presume to measure one or more auditory subskills, few writers offer specific recommendations about tests that might be used in the evaluation process. For example, Semel's Auditory Processing Program (SAPP) (1976) states:

> While there are a number of devices available for screening and testing children with auditory processing problems, there is no single device, as

---

[‡] Available from DLM (Developmental Learning Materials, 7440 Natchez Avenue, Niles, IL 60648).

yet, that can lead to a detailed assessment of all the important areas of language processing. Most individual tests focus on one or just a few auditory skills. Consequently, even the best selection of tests will still pass by a certain percentage of children who will later exhibit severe management difficulties.

Thus, the choice of tests that represent the "best selection" and an estimation of what each measures is left to the individual examiner prior to implementing Semel's remedial program.

Butler (1980) takes a similar position regarding tests of auditory processing. She states, "there are hundreds of tests purporting to measure auditory processing and speech and language skills. The specialist is responsible for selecting the 'most appropriate' tests, taking into account their reliability and validity."

Greater specifics are offered by Rampp (1980), as shown in Table 1, although he acknowledges that his recommended test battery is provided only as a guideline. He includes a list of additional tests in the appendix of his book. Many of the tests listed in Table 1 represent, in our judgment, tests that have less auditory than linguistic content. Therefore, test selection of the type listed would be difficult to prioritize.

Allen, Bliss, and Timmons (1981) illustrate that difficulty in a study that compared three standardized measures of language development with the judgments of three experienced speech-language pathologists. Their results, presented in Table 2, show substantial disagreement between clinician judgments and test results, apparently on the basis of differing criteria of what constitutes normal versus impaired language development in children. Children who failed a given test (and there was little agreement among the results of the three tests used) were not necessarily judged as having impaired language, and the reverse was also true. On the basis of these results, the authors concluded that (1) total agreement is not necessary for a valid language assessment; (2) a child's language status should be based upon a careful review of information from both sources; (3) one type of information may be weighted more heavily than the other for certain children, and (4) the evaluation of impaired language behavior in three-year-old children is more an art than a science at the present time.

For those who desire more guidance in test selection, Ralph Rupp at the University of Michigan has recently assembled updated lists of tests for auditory processing and the functions that they are presumed to measure. [§]

[§]For information, write to Ralph R. Rupp, Ph.D., Professor of Education and Audiology, Speech and Hearing Sciences, University of Michigan, 111 East Catherine Street, Ann Arbor, MI 48109.

Table 1
Diagnostic Test Battery of Auditory Processing*

Discrimination
  Wepman
  Goldman-Fristoe-Woodcock: quiet/noise
  Audiologic data

Memory/Sequence
  ITPA: auditory sequential memory
  Detroit Test of Learning Aptitude: unrelated words, related words
  Stanford-Binet: sentence repetition
  WISC: digit memory

Figure-Ground
  Composite Auditory Perceptual Test (CAPT): Parts 1 and 2
  Kindergarten Auditory Screening Test: speech/noise
  Flowers-Costello Central Auditory Abilities Test: competing messages
  Goldman-Fristoe-Woodcock: quiet/noise

Closure
  ITPA: sound blending, auditory closure
  Kindergarten Auditory Screening Test: phonemic synthesis
  Flowers-Costello: low-pass filtered speech

Association
  ITPA: auditory reception and association

Language Subtests
  Receptive vocabulary: Peabody Picture Vocabulary Test
  Auditory reception: ITPA
  Articulation competency: Goldman-Fristoe, McDonald
  Language Facility Test: spontaneous language

Cognitive/Academic
  Intelligence: WISC, Leiter, Stanford-Binet
  Academic: WRAT
  Concepts: Boehm
  Reading: Gray, Durrell, Gates-MacGinitie

Visual
  Discrimination: Frostig, Bender Visual-Motor Gestalt Test
  Memory/Sequence: ITPA (visual sequential memory), Detroit (objects, letters)
  Association: ITPA (visual reception and association)
  Closure: ITPA (visual closure)
  Integration: Birch A-V Integration

From Rampp D (1980). Auditory processing and learning disabilities, Omaha, Nebraska: Cliff Notes, Inc. With permission.
*Dr. Rampp modifies this outline over time (personal communication).

Table 2
Summary of Decisions by Test and Clinician

Test	N	Percent Language-Impaired by Test	Percent Language-Impaired by Clinician	Percent Language-Impaired by Clinician Judged Normal-Speaking by Test	Percent Language-Impaired by Test Judged Normal-Speaking by Clinician
CELI*	148	14.2	12.2	27.8	38.1
TACL†	149	5.4	14.1	81.0	41.2
SICD‡	171	9.9	15.2	61.5	50.0

From Allen D, Bliss L, & Timmons J (1981). Language evaluation: science or art? *Journal of Speech and Hearing Disorders, 46*, 66–68. With permission.
*CELI—Carrow Elicited Language Inventory
†TACL—Test of Auditory Comprehension of Language
‡SICD—Sequenced Inventory of Communication Development

Both Semel and Rampp have emphasized that, in addition to the administration of formal tests, the diagnostician should take advantage of both observation of the child at play and the case history. We strongly agree. Moreover, many diagnostic findings can be more meaningful in light of case history information. We concur with Rampp that the history is one of the most valuable means of assessing the child, because parents know more about their own child than anyone else. We caution the inexperienced clinician that tests must be accurately and intelligently administered and their results viewed in light of observed behaviors and the case history information. Even then, the conclusions drawn may not account for individual differences in such factors as motivation, compensatory skills, and attention span. Moreover, some authors of auditory tests fail to account for the multitudes of test environment influences that might invalidate the tests, except to caution that the tests should be administered in the "quiet area" of a given facility. Fundamental questions might well be, "How quiet does a quiet room need to be for a given test procedure?" and "Is it consistently quiet, or does the ambient noise level change intermittently?" One would not typically accept an audiologist's results of pure tone and speech audiometry on a patient if such tests were not administered in a sound-treated test booth with carefully calibrated instruments and precisely controlled stimulus intensity levels.

Butler (1980) has diagrammed the model of evaluation of auditory-processing disorders shown in Figure 1. It may be noted that auditory

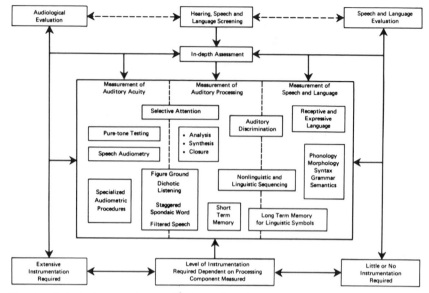

Fig. 1. Selected areas for evaluation of auditory-processing disorders (From Butler, K. (1980) Disorders of other aspects auditory function. In R. VanHattum (Ed.), *Communication disorders.* New York: MacMillan Publishing, 147. With permission.)

discrimination is listed as a function measured in the speech and language assessment, while speech audiometry is listed under measurement of auditory acuity. Others, particularly audiologists, use the term speech audiometry to mean measurements of both speech reception thresholds and speech discrimination. Butler lists both dichotic listening and Staggered Spondaic Words (SSW) under figure-ground tasks. The SSW (Katz, 1968) is, a dichotic listening test. She also lists filtered-speech as another test of figure-ground skill. However, this test utilizes degraded signals and is administered in a controlled, quiet background. Thus it appears to us to be more an auditory closure task. Rampp (1980) lists figure-ground, dichotic listening, the SSW, and filtered-speech merely as specialized audiometric procedures. Wiig and Semel (1976) take still another view. They discuss the SSW under the subtitle of speech reception and speech discrimination. It would appear, from such differences in categorizations, that there is considerable disagreement about what such tests measure.

Sloan (1980) takes a different view of evaluating auditory processing function, stating that there is no test for auditory processing disorders. She cites several kinds of tests that are presented through the ear, such as receptive language tests, auditory language comprehension tests, speech sound discrimination tests, and sound retention tests. However, she adds that none is comprehensive enough to provide a basis for differential diagnosis. She notes further that too many factors enter into any test situation, which contribute to the child's success or failure. Thus, she feels that there is little likelihood that a given test will distinguish a central auditory processing disorder. She believes that the best way to evaluate and diagnose children with central auditory problems is with an assortment of speech and language measures "that focus on different aspects of speech, language, and auditory function." Such a view is common among professionals who see the language-auditory processing relationship as one of clear, straight-forward cause and effect. We suspect that many advertised tests of auditory perceptual skills are really tests of some facet of language function. Sloan apparently agrees, since she defines auditory processing disorders as, "problems in the accurate and efficient transmission of acoustic information important to speech perception; that have a secondary effect on the development of articulation and language as well." Although we do not question that auditory factors do influence language processes, as mentioned earlier, we will show later that there are children who have central auditory processing disorders (CAPD) that are severe enough to have a profound influence on their life, but who do not have significant language deficiencies. Thal (1978), Tallal and Newcombe (1978), Tallal, Stark, Kallman, and Mellits (1980), and Ludlow (1980) have reported similar findings. Whether auditory processing provides the foundation for language or whether it is dependent on language in order to function efficiently is a debatable issue. Perhaps there are both types of processing. An interesting argument for this position has been presented by Duchan and Katz (1983), who propose that "top down" plus "bottom up" factors are involved in language and auditory processing. Butler (1980) suggests the possibility that children who have language processing and attention disorders may well differ in degree, if not kind, in the execution of auditory tasks. Based on substantial clinical data we are convinced that it is a fact rather than a possibility.

Neuropsychological Approach

Neuropsychologists have a fundamental interest in comprehensive brain-behavior relationships (Hynd & Obrzut, 1981), of which they typically take a broad view. In that same source Hynd (1981) reviews evidence to show that estimates of the number of neuropsychological evaluation instruments varies from less than 100 to more than 200, of which the most commonly used are the Wechsler Adult Intelligence Scale, the Bender Visual-Motor Gestalt Test, and the Halstead-Reitan Neuropsychological Test Battery. He cites Craig (1979) for stating that the era of using one test is over, and states that, although there is much validity to neuropsychological batteries and that they are reasonably accurate in determining presence or absence of brain impairment, they are somewhat limited in their ability to detect impaired psychological processes reliably or in determining the site of impairment and the degree of chronicity. Auditory tests are particularly ignored in neuropsychological test batteries. One such battery, the Revised Neurological Key (Aaron, 1981) includes 11 different tests with but a lone measure of sequential memory (Goldman, Fristoe, & Woodcock, 1974) representing the auditory assessment of brain function. In the Reitan-Kløve Sensory Perceptual Examination, the examiner measures auditory perception skill by "lightly rubbing the fingers together very quickly and sharply" (Selz, 1981). In still a third battery, the Halstead Neuropsychological Test Battery for Children, the examiner utilizes a taped series of 60 spoken nonsense words as the measure of speech-sounds perception. It would appear that the above tests may lack the sophistication to identify subtle CANS dysfunction.

A significant number of parents who bring children to our center for evaluation of unexplained social and academic behaviors have been through extensive evaluation by both school speech-language pathologists and psychologists with unremarkable results. One is impelled to speculate about the reasons for this commonly occurring experience. One reason may be that a child's performance on the various diagnostic tests simply failed to meet the specific criteria for identification as LD established by the school district, or by the specific diagnostic team within a given district.[1] Another reason may be that the diagnostic team utilizes tests that lack the sensitivity to identify a subtle deficiency in central auditory function, which may be sufficient to cause the child's social and academic difficulties. Yet, he has no noticeable or significant language or academic deficiency by the diagnostic team's standards. The first reasons suggested could well be prime contributors to the problem, as we have attempted to point out in the preceding discussion. Support for these alternatives may be found in the work of Shephard and Smith (1981) who conducted a large and carefully designed study to evaluate the procedures and results of the identification of children with perceptual-communicative disorders (PCD) in Colorado. PCD is conceptually similar to the federal definition of specific LD, as defined earlier. Their investigation included analyses of referral, assessment, staffing, and placement, and their evaluation of the adequacy of assessment is of particular perti-

---

[1]The Director of Special Education in one large public school system acknowledges that different diagnostic teams within that system do employ different criteria in the diagnostic process, and that it is usually the psychologist, the team leader, who is primarily responsible for that diversity. However, individual professional judgment and choice of test instrument is encouraged.

and their evaluation of the adequacy of assessment is of particular perti-
nence to this discussion. It included surveys of representative samples of
professionals in order to ascertain the beliefs, opinions, and practices of
principals, PCD (i.e., LD) teachers, psychologists, and speech-language
pathologists about PCD identification (Table 3). Their findings are sober-
ing, as the following summary will attest:

1. Variations in the prevalence of PCD among units and across years
    suggest the existence of local patterns of strictness and laxness in the
    identification of PCD.
2. Professionals who participate in the identification of PCD differ
    widely in the extent to which their individual views match the legal
    definition of PCD.
3. Of the 18 most frequently used tests in PCD assessment, only 5 are
    adequate. Most tests used do not have adequate reliability and valid-
    ity. They found this to be especially true of tests for processing
    deficits when compared with achievement and IQ tests. Moreover,
    nearly 50 percent of professionals were unaware of these factors in
    the tests they use.
4. Clinical judgment is frequently cited as an alternative to tests in
    assessment. However, there are few signs that clinical judgment
    improves the validity of PCD identification. Clinical judgments about
    processing disorders were found to be consistent only a small propor-
    tion of the time, and clinicians interpreted single signs as being
    dysfunctions when they are just as frequently found among normal
    children.
5. More than half of the children currently placed in PCD classes do not
    meet *either* statistical or valid clinical criteria for identification of PCD,
    and many of the "non-handicapped" children have serious problems
    in school and need special help.
6. For the 20 to 25 percent of PCD cases who have no signs of a handicap
    or who are not seriously below grade level, it is reasonable to propose
    that the disorder is in the school environment rather than in the child.

Assuming the Shepard and Smith study to be without fault of its own, it
serves as a serious indictment of current diagnostic assessment of children who are frequently assigned the label of LD as a result of having an
assumed processing deficit. Still further evidence of inadequacies of
diagnostic tests has been reported by Thurlow and Ysseldyke (1970), as
shown in Table 4. On the basis of our experience, several of the foregoing
factors may lie at fault. However, we have found that an imposing
number of these children have CAPD, which has gone previously undi-
agnosed. An interesting facet of this situation is that the finding of a
CAPD often squares with teacher and parent reports in the case history

Table 3

Percents of PCD Teachers, School Psychologists, and Speech/Language Specialists Reporting Frequency of use and Judgments about Reliability and Validity.*

| | Frequency of Use | | | | | Reliability & Validity* | | | | | |
| | | | | | | Reliability | | | Validity | | |
	Never 0%	Rarely 1–15%	Sometimes 16–50%	Often 51–85%	Nearly Always 86–100%	1	2	3	1	2	3
					PCD Teachers						
Detroit Tests of Learning Aptitude[†]	20	16	18	15	16	39	17	15	32	19	18
Peabody Picture Vocabulary Test (PPVT)	19	19	17	13	16	47	14	10	41	15	10
Woodcock-Johnson Psychoeducational Battery	28	3	8	12	35	60	3	9	56	3	8
KeyMath Diagnostic Arithmetic Test	7	10	23	26	21	60	4	7	58	5	8
Peabody Individual Achievement Tests (PIAT)	10	12	13	16	35	40	23	8	38	22	9
Wide Range Achievement Test (WRAT)	16	12	21	15	20	35	24	10	30	25	12
Woodcock Reading Mastery Tests	19	11	15	18	20	49	6	12	45	6	13
Beery Developmental Test of Visual-Motor Integration (VMI)	15	9	15	14	32	49	10	10	46	10	11
					School Psychologists						
WISC-R	0	5	9	29	54	89	3	1	85	6	1
Wide Range Achievement Test (WRAT)	20	15	30	16	11	49	20	14	40	30	13
Draw-a-Person (Goodenough-Harris Drawing Test)	8	16	16	23	34	45	31	8	45	30	10

Test											
Kinetic Family Drawing	8	18	25	26	15	32	33	12	30	33	13
Sentence Completion	6	20	32	28	11	32	32	20	36	28	18
Beery Developmental Test of Visual-Motor Integration (VMI)	24	21	14	19	14	55	11	14	48	17	14
Bender (Visual-Motor) Gestalt Test	5	11	13	22	48	64	11	8	57	18	7
Speech Language Specialists											
Detroit Tests of Learning Aptitude	7	15	24	24	21	52	20	6	45	22	10
Peabody Picture Vocabulary Test (PPVT)	2	6	7	21	58	65	13	6	59	14	8
WISC-R	43	2	7	12	19	48	3	11	47	4	10
Spencer Memory for Sentences Test	16	18	20	17	10	29	22	15	27	21	17
Wepman Auditory Discrimination Test (The Wepman)	6	13	29	23	20	39	31	8	34	30	10
Boehm Test of Basic Concepts	8	18	24	29	13	68	5	5	64	6	4
Carrow Tests for Auditory Comprehension of Language	3	7	27	36	23	77	3	3	70	4	5
Goldman-Fristoe Test of Articulation	22	14	17	21	19	63	2	7	57	3	7
Illinois Test of Psycholinguistic Abilities (ITPA)	13	23	25	21	11	47	20	7	39	21	11

From Shepard L & Smith M (1981). Evaluation of the identification of perceptual communicative disorders. Laboratory of Educational Research, Department of Education, University of Colorado. With permission.

*A longer list of tests was included on the original questionnaire.

*1 = Adequate; 2 = Inadequate; 3 = Don't Know.

†Tests are included here if more than 40 percent of any group said they used it "with more than half of the children they assessed."

Table 4

Ratings of the Technical Adequacy of Devices Used
Nationally in Child Service Demonstration Centers[a]

	Norms	Reliability	Validity
Beery Developmental Test of Visual-Motor Integration	−	−	−
Bender Visual-Motor Gestalt	−	−	−
Brigance Inventory of Basic Skills	−	−	−
California Test of Basic Skills	*	*	*
Carrow Elicited Language Inventory	−	−	−
Detroit Tests of Learning Aptitude	−	−	−
Gates-McKillop Reading Diagnostic Tests	−	−	−
Gilmore Oral Reading Test	−	−	−
Goldman-Fristoe Test of Articulation	CR[b]	+	+
Illinois Test of Psycholinguistic Abilities	−	−	−
KeyMath Diagnostic Arithmetic Test[c]	−	−	−
McCarthy Scales of Children's Abilities	+	+	+
Motor Free Visual Perception	−	−	−
Peabody Individual Achievement Tests[c]	+	+	+
Peabody Picture Vocabulary Test	−	+	+
Piers-Harris Self-Concept Scale	−	−	−
Ruben	*	*	*
Slossen	−	−	−
SRA Achievement	+	−	−
Spache Diagnostic Reading Scales	−	−	−
Stanford Achievement Test	+	+	+
Stanford-Binet	+	−	−
Test for Auditory Comprehension	+	−	−
Utah Test of Language Development	−	−	−
Wepman Auditory Discrimination Test	−	−	−
WAIS	+	+	+
WISC-R[c]	+	+	+
Wide Range Achievement Test[c]	−	+	−
Woodcock-Johnson Psycho-Educational Battery	+	+	+
Woodcock Reading Mastery	+	+	+

From Thurlow M & Ysseldyke J (1979). Current assessment and decision-making practices in model LD programs. *Learning Disability Quarterly, 2,* 15–24. With permission.
[a] + = technically adequate.
  − = technically inadequate.
  * = manual not available.
[b] Test is criterion-referenced.
[c] Devices used by more than half of all responding centers (N = 39).

and frequently with the child's testimony as well, e.g., complains about inability to hear the teacher, the other kids making too much noise, or other factors in the classroom that interfere with ability to attend. The same kinds of difficulties are experienced in the home when the parent speaks to the child from a different room or from a different floor of the house, often with a television, stereo, or radio playing or an appliance running. Rampp (1980) cautions that some diagnosticians may fail to recognize that mothers know more about their children than anyone else. As a result, historical information is often poorly integrated into the evaluation process. Thus, the history is a critical instrument to support test performance and clinical judgment, regardless of whether the outcome leads to therapeutic intervention or simply to modifications in the child's academic and social environments.

In summary, it appears that we may be working with imperfect assessment tools and with limited knowledge of the events in human auditory function. It appears that we may be ignoring central auditory function per se. Therefore, it is our position that we need to determine the child's problem through an appropriate case history and then assess his central auditory function and other brain-behavior functions with techniques that place enough stress on the CANS to reveal an abnormality that would account for the concerns revealed in the case history.

Audiological Approach

Audiologists have traditionally taken a different approach to assessing CAPD. Bocca and Calearo (1963) presented a comprehensive summary of audiologic methods for diagnosing disorders in the CANS, methods that sought simply to define the site of neuroaudiologic lesions as opposed, except in the case of aphasic persons, to studying the behavioral impact of such lesions. The development of tests for this purpose, however, was strongly influenced by knowledge of the nature of sensory aphasia and its relationship to language processes. Nonetheless, audiologic attention was focused on supporting neurologic diagnoses of adult patients with CANS insults, which constituted a potential threat to life. Such interest has continued to the present time (Brunt, 1978; Hurley, 1980; Jerger, 1973; Lynn & Gilroy, 1976, 1977; Noffsinger & Kurdziel, 1979; and numerous others). Although the use of audiologic tests supplemented traditional diagnostic procedures, the purpose of the tests and control of the patient remained the responsibility of medical specialists.

In the 1970s interest began to develop in the use of central auditory tests with children (Beasley & Rintelmann, 1979; Lasky & Katz, 1983; McCroskey & Kasten, 1980; Willeford & Billger, 1978; and others). In this development, however, the concern was no longer focused on identifying lesions in the CANS for medical purposes. Rather, these efforts involved children in whom there was concern about academic and social deficiencies and, in some instances, an accompanying language disorder. The audiological approach with CAPD children was primarily to define the functional status of their CANS to provide better insights into their management as addressed in Chapter 6.

In the writers' perspective, audiological tests of central auditory processing (CAP) measure "auditory channel capacity," or the intactness, integrity (functional status), or fundamental efficiency of the CANS by subjecting it to "difficult" auditory listening tasks. In other words, the CANS performance is tested under "auditory stress" conditions. The test results correlate with practical auditory processes necessary for efficient social functioning (including the academic classroom) that places a premium on correct interpretation of auditory signals in one's environment. They do not necessarily imply that poor performance means that an individual has either a language problem or a learning disability by legal and professional definitions, although some do have one or both. It does mean, however, that school achievement and social success is difficult for them, that they must work harder to get the same information as non-CAPD children, and that they will perform below their level of potential in life. The impact on their psychological makeup is often substantial, as discussed in Chapter 7, to the degree that it appears to contribute to social rejection and even to juvenile delinquency in some instances.

2

The Auditory System

The accurate processing of auditory information involves a complex sequence of neurophysiological events that require the integrated functions of both the peripheral and central nervous systems. Each plays a vital role in the process of transmitting audible vibratory energy from the environment into an ultimately meaningful experience to the receiver. Because of this, the auditory system is one of the most fascinating parts of the human body. Given adequate sensory reception, auditory signals must pass through an elaborate series of neural processes and specialized nerve fibers and cellular structures that permit a progressively refined analysis of the signal as it moves through this unique system.

PERIPHERAL AUDITORY SYSTEM

The peripheral hearing mechanism is a system that is separable into four main sections: (1) outer ear; (2) middle ear; (3) inner ear, and (4) eighth cranial nerve (Fig. 2).

The outer ear, comprised of the auricle and the external auditory meatus, is chiefly regarded for its ability to collect and convey sound vibrations to the middle ear system. The external meatus also functions as a protective mechanism for the middle ear by virtue of its location, shape, cilia, and production of cerumen. It also acts as a resonator of sound in the frequency region of about 3800 Hz, however, this resonating frequency may vary according to the size and shape of the external auditory meatus (Zemlin, 1968).

Sound waves are then transmitted via vibratory movement of the tympanic membrane to the middle ear cavity, which contains the ossicular chain, stapedius muscle, tensor tympani muscle, seventh cranial nerve (facial), and the eustachian tube. Basically, the middle ear serves as a transformer that facilitates the transmission of acoustic energy to the fluid in the inner ear. It decreases the impedance mismatch between the

Gross division	Outer ear	Middle ear	Inner ear	Central auditory nervous system
Anatomy	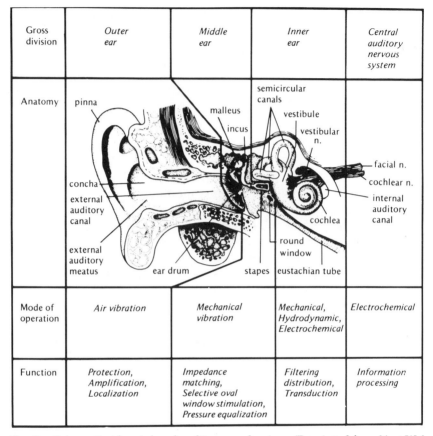			
Mode of operation	Air vibration	Mechanical vibration	Mechanical, Hydrodynamic, Electrochemical	Electrochemical
Function	Protection, Amplification, Localization	Impedance matching, Selective oval window stimulation, Pressure equalization	Filtering distribution, Transduction	Information processing

Fig. 2. Schematic of peripheral auditory mechanism. (Reprinted from Yost W & Nielsen D (1977). *Fundamentals of Hearing*. New York: Holt, Rinehart, & Winston. p. 33. With permission.)

outer ear and the cochlea, thus minimizing the loss of energy in the transmission process. This is necessary because the movement generated at the larger surface of the tympanic membrane must be transmitted to the smaller surface of the oval window without a loss of energy. Also, the actions of the tympanic membrane and the ossicular chain are important in their leverage properties which prepare acoustic energy for entering the inner ear (Zemlin, 1968; Zwislocki, 1975).

The inner ear houses the following sensory organs: utricle, saccule, semicircular canals, and cochlea (Fig. 3). The utricle, saccule, and semi-circular canals serve the important vestibular functions of equilibrium and orientation in space, whereas the cochlea is the primary sensory

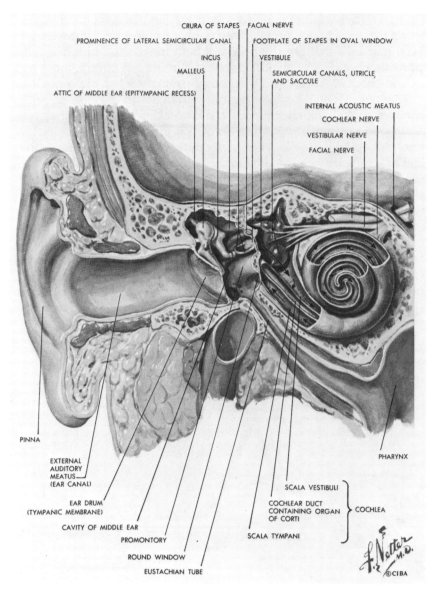

CRURA OF STAPES   FACIAL NERVE

PROMINENCE OF LATERAL SEMICIRCULAR CANAL   FOOTPLATE OF STAPES IN OVAL WINDOW

INCUS   VESTIBULE

MALLEUS   SEMICIRCULAR CANALS, UTRICLE, AND SACCULE

ATTIC OF MIDDLE EAR (EPITYMPANIC RECESS)

INTERNAL ACOUSTIC MEATUS

COCHLEAR NERVE

VESTIBULAR NERVE

FACIAL NERVE

PINNA

PHARYNX

EXTERNAL AUDITORY MEATUS (EAR CANAL)

SCALA VESTIBULI

EAR DRUM (TYMPANIC MEMBRANE)

COCHLEAR DUCT CONTAINING ORGAN OF CORTI   COCHLEA

CAVITY OF MIDDLE EAR

SCALA TYMPANI

PROMONTORY

ROUND WINDOW

EUSTACHIAN TUBE

Fig. 3. Illustration of the peripheral auditory and vestibular system (Reprinted from Netter F (1962a). *Otologic diagnosis and treatment of deafness.* In Meyers D, Schlosser W, Winchester A (Eds.), Summit, NJ: CIBA Pharmaceutical Co. p. 42 With permission.)

23

organ for the reception of auditory stimuli. The cochlea houses the organ of Corti, which contains the sensory receptor cells that are fundamental to all auditory functions (Fig. 4). This mechanism houses approximately 23,000 hair cells that are comprised of both inner and outer hair cells. Approximately 40–60 short cilia project from the top of each inner hair cell, and about 40–120 longer cilia protrude from the top of each outer hair cell (Zemlin, 1968). They are typically arranged in a W shape when viewed from their superior aspect. The longer cilia of the outer hair cells are embedded in a gelatinous mass known as the tectorial membrane that projects over the hair cells. The shorter inner hair cells and some shorter outer hair cells are free-standing in the fluid space (Stillman, 1980). It has been theorized by Bekesy (1960) that the floor of the scala media, or basilar membrane, and the tectorial membrane move in unison when displaced to create a shearing force that impinges on the hair cells and thereby initiates neural impulses, an idea that is now well supported.

The hair cells send impulses to the central nervous system (afferent or sensory neurons) and also receive impulses traveling from the central nervous system (efferent or motor neurons) (Glattke, 1978; Zemlin, 1968). These impulses travel via a bundle of nerve fibers known as the acoustic (VIII cranial) nerve. Fibers from the cochlea travel to the VIIIth nerve via

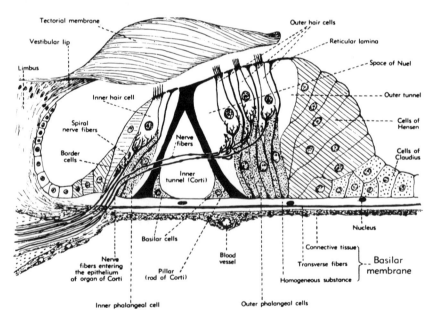

Fig. 4. Illustration of the organ of Corti, including inner and outer hair cells (Reprinted from Rasmussen A, (1943). Outlines of neuro-anatomy. Dubuque, Iowa: W. C. Brown. p. 406. With permission.)

the perforate habenula, an osseous plate located inferior to the organ of Corti. According to Zemlin (1968), the majority of inner hair cells are innervated by more than one nerve fiber and vice versa. The few afferent nerve fibers that extend to the outer hair cells are the outer spiral fibers, which synapse with other hair cells along their route to the outer hair cells. The cell bodies of the neurons that innervate the inner and outer hair cells form a structure called the spiral ganglion, a concentration of cell bodies that is housed in the modiolus (Zemlin, 1968). The latter is shown in Figure 5.

The efferent system is comprised of approximately 500 nerve fibers that terminate primarily at the outer hair cells. However, the remainder follow a route inferior to the inner hair cells and connect with the afferent fibers that are coursing from the inner hair cells (Glattke, 1978). The internal fibers pass through the modiolus and group together to form the auditory section of the VIIIth cranial nerve.

The VIIIth cranial nerve consists of fibers arising from both the cochlear and vestibular systems. It is comprised of approximately 50,000 nerve fibers (Rasmussen, 1940), of which approximately 25,000 (Glattke, 1978) to 31,500 (Zemlin, 1968) individual nerve fibers combine to form the vestibular branch. These fibers pass to the internal acoustic meatus where they separate via a bony shelf known as the transverse crest. The cochlear and saccular branches travel below the transverse crest, whereas the remainder of vestibular fibers are located above this bony shelf. Also passing through the internal acoustic meatus are fibers from the facial (VIIth cranial) nerve, along with fibers from intermediate nerves and blood vessels. After emerging from the internal acoustic meatus these fibers rejoin the cochlear branch of the acoustic nerve and the cochlear bundle and journey directly to the cochlear nucleus in the brainstem. It is interesting to note that the acoustic nerve is relatively short, measuring only five millimeters in length (Zemlin, 1968).

CENTRAL AUDITORY NERVOUS SYSTEM

Cochlear Nucleus

There is general agreement that the CANS functionally begins at the point where the auditory nerve synapses at the cochlear nucleus, where all cochlear nerve fibers have been found to terminate (Fig. 6). Secondary neurons are then projected to various higher levels of the CANS. The cochlear nucleus, located on each side of the brainstem in the region of the medulla, is divided into three primary regions: the dorsal nucleus and the anteroventral and posteroventral nuclei. All cochlear fibers supply

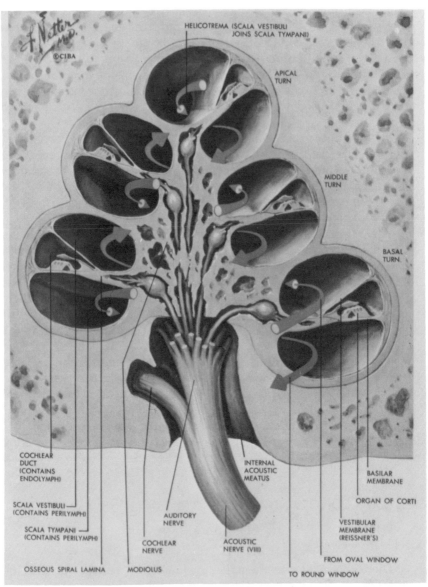

Fig. 5. Cross-section of cochlea (Reprinted from Netter F (1962a). *Otologic diagnosis and treatment of deafness.* In Meyers D, Schlosser W, Winchester A (Eds.), Summit, NJ: CIBA Pharmaceutical Co. p. 43. With permission.)

26

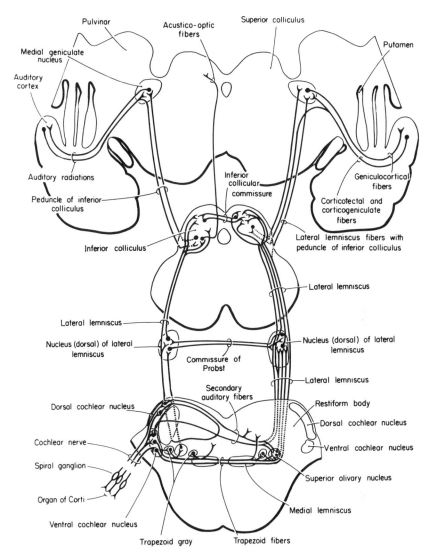

Fig. 6. Illustration of central auditory pathway (Reprinted from Crosby E, Humphrey T, & Lauer E (1962). *Correlative anatomy of the nervous system*. New York: MacMillan. p. 276. With permission.)

branches that ipsilaterally interconnect with each of these subdivisions. Nonetheless, there is evidence that cells in these regions of the cochlear nuclei function in ways that provide a rich variety of responses from auditory signals supplied by the cochlea where initial analyses have been made of frequency and intensity (Kiang, 1975). It appears to be the initial stage of "central processing," the sorting and integrating functions assigned to the coding of auditory signals.

Tonotopic organization is also monitored by an orderly correspondence between regions of the cochlea and sectors of the cochlear nucleus, and a similar correspondence in the ascending pathways preserves selective frequency representation throughout the higher centers (Morest, 1975). A schematic drawing of the spatial distribution of cochlear nerve fibers in the cochlear nucleus is shown in Figure 7. Considerable enlightenment of brainstem functions has also been provided by the research of Kiang (1975), who has demonstrated that different cells in the cochlear nucleus respond in an intriguingly differential manner. Figure 8 demonstrates this phenomenon in the response of five selected cell types to short tone bursts. Kiang uses this figure to illustrate evidence that neural units having characteristic discharge patterns are located in specific regions occupied by known types of cells in the cochlear nucleus. This illustration is limited to five examples of large cell types, although he believes there are many different kinds of cells clustered throughout the

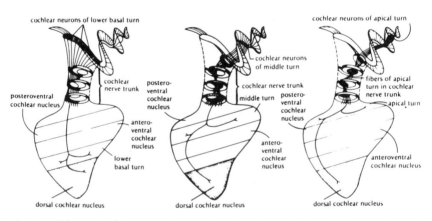

Fig. 7. Schematic diagrams showing that basal turn (left), middle turn (center), and apical turn (right) auditory nerve fibers innervate different areas of the three main regions of the cochlear nucleus. The spatial separation of frequency from base to apex in the cochlea is reflected in the characteristic frequencies of the fibers that leave the cochlea and is maintained within each of the three main regions of the cochlear nucleus (Reprinted from Yost W, & Nielsen D (1977). *Fundamentals of Hearing.* New York: Holt, Rinehart, & Winston. p. 96. With permission.)

CELLS IN THE COCHLEAR NUCLEUS

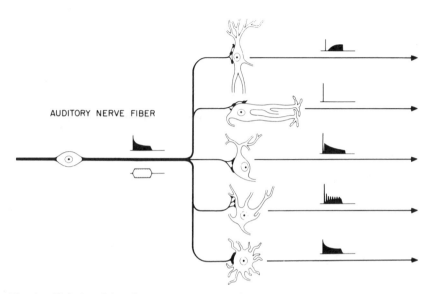

AUDITORY NERVE FIBER

Fig. 8. Relationship of response types in the cochlear nucleus to cell types. A diagrammatic representation of unit types as defined by typical responses to moderate intensity, short (25- to 50-msec) tone bursts at the CF (critical frequency) and the cell types to which the unit types are believed to correspond. This figure should be thought of as a section of Fig. 9 showing a high-CF auditory-nerve fiber and its projections to certain cells in the cochlear nucleus. The PST histogram above the auditory-nerve fiber shows its typical response pattern to tone bursts. The envelope of one tone burst is shown below the fiber. The histograms on the right are typical of unit types that are in order from top to bottom: 1. "Pauser"; 2. "On"; 3. "Primarylike with notch"; 4. "Chopper"; and 5. "Primarylike." For low-Cf units, there is time-locking to individual cycles of the tones; however, the envelopes of the histograms will, in most cases, still resemble those of high-CF units (Reprinted from Kiang N (1975). Stimulus representation in the discharge patterns of auditory neurons. In Eagles, E (Ed.), *The Nervous System*, Vol. 3. New York: Raven Press, p. 89. With permission.)

nucleus. It can be seen in this figure that when short tone bursts are employed as stimuli, some cochlear nucleus cells ("primarylike") respond in a manner essentially like those of auditory nerve fibers. These units are located primarily in the rostral (upper) part of the anteroventral nucleus. In sharp contrast are the "on" units that are predominantly limited to the octopus cell region of the posterior posteroventral cochlear nucleus. A helpful illustration of these cellular arrangements and their relationships to both cochlear nucleus regions and cochlear connections is shown in Figure 9.

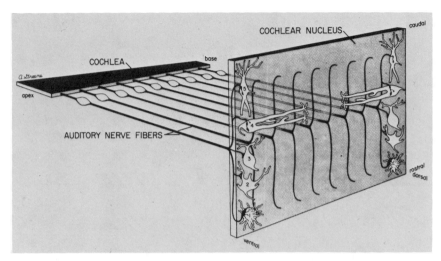

Fig. 9. Schematic representation of anatomical relationships of auditory-nerve fibers to selected cochlear nucleus cells. Since the cochlear nucleus does not actually have the shape of a slab, the directional labels indicate only a general orientation and should not be taken literally. The peripheral extensions of auditory-nerve cells are shown systematically innervating the cochlea in a punctate manner (as in fact the radial fibers do). The central extensions of these cells branch in the cochlear nucleus to innervate many different kinds of cells (five examples shown). Inputs to these cells from the central nervous system are not shown (adapted from Kiang N (1975). Stimulus representation in the discharge patterns of auditory neurons. In Eagles, E (Ed.), *The Nervous System*, Vol. 3. New York: Raven Press, p. 88. With permission.)

Kiang (1975) states that cells of a particular type in the cochlear nucleus project to other specific locations in the brainstem up to the inferior colliculus, but not beyond that point. He uses the illustration in Figure 10 to show this sophisticated network and states that, while such diagrams may appear too complicated to be useful, it is this very complexity that encourages systematic attempts to account for the richness of behavioral responses. He has defined the boundaries of the brainstem as approximately the inconclusive area from the cochlear nucleus to the inferior colliculus, which is the last point of crossover connections between the two lateral lemniscus tracts.

Although it does not supply specific references or documentation, the Report of the Panel on Communicative Disorders (1979) summarizes the state of knowledge concerning the cochlear nucleus. It confirms Kiang's work and concludes that such information is essential to an interpretation of studies of the response properties of cells in this complex

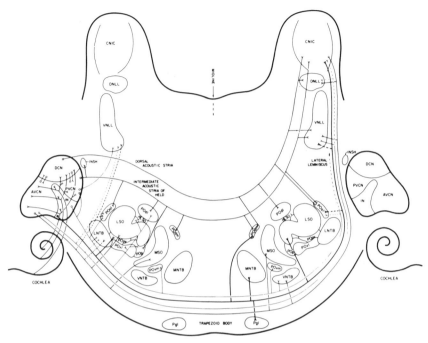

Fig. 10. Schematic diagram of anatomically described output pathways of the cochlear nucleus. The cochlea is represented by a spiral, the cochlear nucleus by an idealized sagittal section, the medulla by an idealized transverse section, and the inferior colliculus by an idealized transverse section in a more rostral plane. Solid lines—pathways considered to be well documented; dotted lines—pathways for which some evidence exists, but not of a conclusive nature. To simplify the drawing, the pathways are not strictly correct in all anatomic details (such as the relative position of various fiber components in the trapezoid body). AVCN, anteroventral cochlear nucleus; CNIC, central nucleus of the inferior colliculus; DCN, dorsal cochlear nucleus; DNLL, dorsal nucleus of the lateral lemniscus; HLSO, dorsal hilus of the lateral superior olivary nucleus; IN, interstitial nucleus of the cochlear nucleus; INSH, interstitial nucleus of the stria of Held; LNTB, lateral nucleus of the trapezoid body; LSO, lateral superior olivary nucleus; MNTB, medial nucleus of the trapezoid body; MSO, medial superior olivary nucleus; Pgl, lateral paragigantocellular nucleus; POal, anterolateral periolivary nucleus; POdl, dorsolateral periolivary nucleus; POdm, dorsomedial periolivary nucleus; POp, posterior periolivary nucleus; POpv, posteroventral periolivary nucleus; POvl, ventrolateral periolivary nucleus; POvm, ventromedial periolivary nucleus; PVCN, posteroventral cochlear nucleus; VNLL, ventral nucleus of the lateral lemniscus; VNTB, ventral nucleus of the trapezoid body (Reprinted from Kiang N (1975). Stimulus representation in the discharge patterns of auditory neurons. In Eagles E (Ed.), *The Nervous System*, Vol. 3. New York: Raven Press, p. 92. With permission.)

nucleus. The report further states that the technology for learning the anatomical and neurochemical connection of cell classes is now available, and suggests that these connections may serve different functions and will provide some of the most interesting studies in physiology in the near future. Such research may shed new light in particular on subtle CANS disorders. It may help to establish to what degree cell functions in the cochlear nucleus must be altered before behavioral functions are impaired.

Kiang (1975) questions the minimum number of cells that must be activated in the system to provide useful hearing. The variety of output terminations of the cochlear nucleus no doubt reflects the diversity of behavioral responses that possibly result from sound stimulation. Specific responses such as middle-ear reflexes, arousal responses, pitch and loudness judgments, sound localization, and speech discrimination may be mediated by chains of neurons that are presently definable.

He points out that it is not essential that all of these functions be restored for certain processes to be regained. He cites as examples: (1) hearing aids that are useful even though they obviously do not afford normal hearing, and (2) recognition of the speaker by the listener without the necessity for localization. Thus, it may be that only certain parts of the CANS need to be activated for useful hearing to result. Conversely, we would point out, it may be that if only certain parts of the CANS can be activated, under what listening circumstances does it constitute a limitation in social functions? When does it impair the full and efficient functioning necessary to perform adequately in complex auditory environments such as the classroom, especially an "open" classroom, when the individual's hearing in quiet environments is adequate?

It is the latter skill that raises our concern for children with central auditory disorders. They may be representative of the individuals Kiang (1975) was referring to when he wrote, "It is well established that intentional lesions in animals and naturally occurring neurological defects in humans can affect performance in some auditory tasks without impairing other aspects of hearing." He suggests that neurons that take part in the stapedial reflex would not show the same response characteristics as neurons involved in sound localization. The same appears to be true for binaural stimulation of the auditory system such as occurs with tests of masking level differences and binaural fusion, and tests that require the extraction of embedded signals or the synthesizing of signals sequentially alternating between the two ears. Our discussion of clinical data will offer supporting evidence that this may well be the case. According to Stillman (1980), cochlear nucleus processing takes place in the cell bodies, triggered by action potentials that release a chemical transmitter that directs a flow of ions into the cell. This action produces a temporary electrical charge in the cell membrane, which may cause either an excitatory or an inhibitory potential. When the sum of these potentials exceeds a threshold at some point in time, an action potential is generated and transmitted along the axon. If their sum fails to exceed that threshold, however, no action potential occurs. Therefore, action potentials depend on the summation of inputs from several sources and may be blocked by inhibitory input from several sources. Thus, the timing of inputs to neurons will determine whether they respond (excitatory sum) or are prevented from responding (inhibitory sum). This feature, when combined with multiple innervation and differential firing characteristics of diverse neurons, provides an incalculable variety of response capabilities that seem necessary in order to encode complex stimuli like speech, especially when received in unfavorable acoustic environments or imbedded in competing ambient signals. Moreover, Stillman also asserts that initial sound analysis is demonstrated by the fact that the temporal features of a sound are exhibited in the response of cochlear nucleus neurons. The importance of temporal resolution in the response is to establish a pattern of neural firing that makes possible the distribution of stimulus information through appropriate neural channels via the post-synaptic integration process. He further states that the precise timing of excitatory and inhibitory inputs to each cell along the auditory pathway is critical if each cell is to respond only when the appropriate environmental sound is present. Such a detailed discussion of the cochlear nuclei may seem excessive, but we believe it is justified in order to establish proper respect for central nervous system events that should be included in the concept of auditory processing. While, as stated earlier, there is no doubt that audition is intimately linked to linguistic behaviors, that relationship is still very poorly understood. Thus, the terms "auditory processing" or "auditory perception" in relation to language and/or learning disorders should be used with care.

Superior Olivary Complex

The majority of the fibers from the cochlear nucleus decussate and may terminate in the trapezoid body, the superior olivary complex, or the reticular activating system (Carpenter, 1972). Some of the fibers leaving the ventral cochlear nucleus terminate in the medial and lateral nuclei of the superior olive on the same side, but the majority of the fibers that form the system of the trapezoid body cross to the opposite side and synapse in the nuclei of the trapezoid body and superior olivary complex from which the lateral lemniscus arises (Baru & Karaseva, 1972). However, some fibers of the trapezoid body are not interrupted in the superior olivary complex. Rather, they project directly to the lateral lemniscus and terminate in its nuclei and in the inferior colliculus, while solitary fibers may also terminate in the medial geniculate bodies. This intricate arrangement is illustrated in Figure 11. Furthermore, collaterals from the cells of the trapezoid body run to the nuclei of the sixth cranial (abducens) nerve and cells of the reticular activating system and the motor nucleus of the fifth cranial (trigeminal) nerve (Baru & Karaseva 1972). Thus, auditory complexities of the cochlear nucleus are further compounded by the elaborate neuron connections in the superior olivary complex. Not only is this mechanism an important relay station of the ascending tract, but it also plays a unique role in the elaborate system that provides for binaural listening capabilities. It is intimately involved in the cross-correlation behaviors of the two ears that afford us the selective listening skills we enjoy in group conversations such as the committee meeting, the cocktail party, and the classroom discussion. An example of this action is again provided in Figure 12, which illustrates the input productions to two types of cells in the superior olivary complex that respond to acoustic signals from either ear. It has been shown, however, that signals from the two ears must have synchronized arrival times for binaural cells to be activated. Thus, a delayed signal from one ear would negate a binaural response. Such may be the case for CAPD children.

Lateral Lemniscus

The lateral lemniscus is the primary auditory pathway in the brainstem. It contains fibers arising bilaterally from the superior olivary complex and trapezoid nuclei, most of which terminate in the inferior colliculus. The two lateral lemnisci are also connected by Probst's commissure, located just rostral to the superior olivary complex, the functional significance of which is moot and the existence of which is seldom even mentioned in neurological texts. It is generally agreed that the lateral lemnisci are simply transmission lines for ascending and descending fibers through the brainstem.

Inferior Colliculus

From the lateral lemniscus, the vast majority of fibers progress to the inferior colliculus. Whitfield (1967) reported early research by Cajal in 1909, which suggested that the inferior colliculus and the medial geniculate body receive bifurcated fibers from the lateral lemniscus. However, current observations have revealed that the majority of fibers departing from the lateral lemnisci terminate in the inferior colliculus. New fibers then originate from the inferior colliculus, which proceed to the medial geniculate body.

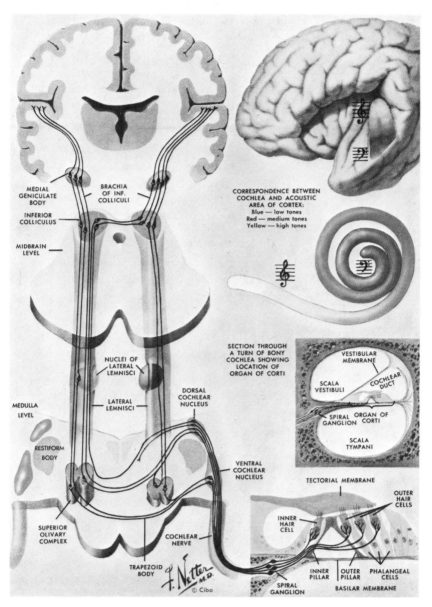

Fig. 11.   Schematic of central auditory nervous system (Reprinted from Netter F (1962b). *Nervous System*. Summit, NJ: CIBA Pharmaceutical Co. p. 64. With permission.)

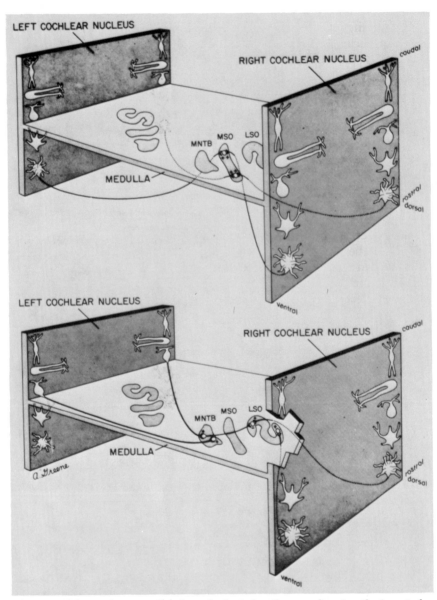

Fig. 12. Schematic representation of selected pathways showing the inputs for two types of units in the superior olivary complex that respond to acoustic stimulation of both ears (Reprinted from Kiang N (1975). Stimulus representation in the discharge patterns of auditory neurons. In Eagles E (Ed.), *The Nervous System*, Vol. 3. New York: Raven Press, p. 94. With permission.)

36

Structurally,* the inferior colliculus is divided into two main parts, the central nucleus and the external nucleus. Investigators (Goldberg & Moore, 1967; Woolard & Harpman, 1940) have observed that the majority of fibers coursing from the lateral lemniscus terminate at the central nucleus of the inferior colliculus. The inferior colliculus also receives ascending fibers from the cochlear nucleus and the superior olivary complex. Tonotopical organization has been better defined for the main central nucleus than for the external nucleus (Rose, Greenwood, Goldberg, & Hind, 1963). The inferior colliculus also receives descending information from the auditory cortex, and it is speculated that transmission is received from the medial geniculate body (Report of the Panel on Communicative Disorders, 1979).

Although the different functions of the inferior colliculus have not been fully ascertained, some evidence suggests that this nucleus represents the highest level of tonotopic organization of neurons for tonal discrimination in the auditory pathways (Whitfield, 1967). Another alleged function of the inferior colliculus is facilitation of binaural localization of both low and high frequencies. Although an abundance of research supporting this premise has not been recorded, Rose, Gross, Geisler, and Hind (1966) have documented the phenomenon.

Erulkar (1959) reported that although the inferior colliculus was organized in tonotopic fashion, not all of its neural units responded to pure tone stimuli. Some of the units responded only to clicks. Unfortunately, responses to complex stimuli were not reported. Rose et al (1963) later provided other details on the firing patterns of the various neurons in the inferior colliculus. Many different patterns were recorded, even from successive, identical stimuli. Hind, Goldberg, Greenwood, and Rose (1963) observed that stimulation of the neurons in one ear produced either a reduced response or an absence of response when simultaneous stimuli were presented to the opposite ear. It would seem that this action would also influence sound localization, but that has not been confirmed, and there are still many unanswered questions regarding the specific involvement of the inferior colliculus in sound localization. However, it may have important implications for a better understanding of certain central auditory tests and of central auditory disorders and their management. In terms of function, it seems obvious that the inferior colliculus is instrumental in serving as a relay center for conveying auditory information to thalamic levels (Carpenter, 1972).

---

*The majority of research concerning the structure of the inferior colliculus has involved the use of various animals such as the monkey, cat, and guinea pig (Barnes, Magoun, & Ranson, 1943; Goldberg & Moore, 1967; Rasmussen, 1946; Woolard & Harpman, 1940).

Medial Geniculate Body

The medial geniculate body appears to be made up of different types of substructures that are structurally diversified (Brodal, 1969; Report of the Panel on Communicative Disorders, 1979). The anatomical structure and the organization of the medial geniculate body are highly complex and a great deal remains unknown about this mechanism. However, studies have shown that they are made up of a small-celled central division called the *pars principalis* and a large-celled division referred to as the *pars magnocellularis* (Brodal, 1969; Whitfield, 1967). According to Rose and Woolsey (1949), the small-celled principal division appears to be the only *auditory* area of the medial geniculate body. Morest (1964) has divided the medial geniculate body into more minute sections and clearly confirmed that these structures are very intricately organized. For example, he found that the fibers of the inferior colliculus terminate primarily in the laminated ventral section of the nucleus. From the ventral section of the medial geniculate body, the fibers project upward to the superior temporal gyrus section of the temporal lobes (Brodal, 1969; Report of the Panel on Communicative Disorders, 1979). Morest (1964) also believes that the medial geniculate body receives projections from the spinal cord that are received in the medial portion of the nucleus. Moreover, the pars magnocellularis seems to be related to the transmission of somatosensory impulses (Brodal, 1969). This mechanism receives descending fibers from the cerebral cortex, including, perhaps, its nonauditory sections (Report of the Panel on Communicative Disorders, 1979).

Functionally, the medial geniculate body appears to be tonotopically organized and, as such, is important in the transmission of particular frequency information to the cortex. When compared with the inferior colliculus, however, the tonotopic organization is much more limited, and some researchers suggest that it is not critical for tonal discrimination (Whitfield, 1967). The medial geniculate body comprises the highest level of subcortical recoding prior to transmission to the cortex. It has also been reported that this mechanism maintains information for localization mainly by its reception of binaural stimuli (Report of the Panel on Communicative Disorders, 1979). It is unfortunate that, because of its subcortical location, the medial geniculate body cannot be analyzed visually, and electrophysiological studies are more difficult to implement.

Reticular Activating System

The reticular formation, or reticular activating system, is a complex neural mechanism located in the central core of the brainstem (Fig. 13).

Moruzzi and Magoun (1949) report that the reticular activating system is involved in altering the level of consciousness and in sustaining the

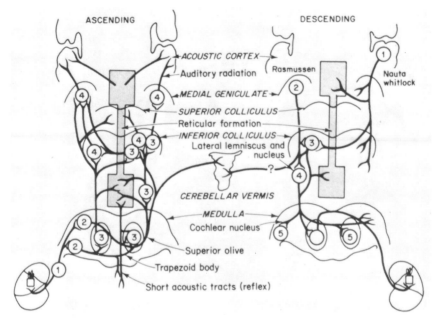

ASCENDING DESCENDING

ACOUSTIC CORTEX
Auditory radiation
Rasmussen
Nauta whitlock
MEDIAL GENICULATE
SUPERIOR COLLICULUS
Reticular formation
INFERIOR COLLICULUS
Lateral lemniscus and nucleus
?
CEREBELLAR VERMIS
MEDULLA
Cochlear nucleus
Superior olive
Trapezoid body
Short acoustic tracts (reflex)

Fig. 13. Schematic of central auditory pathways including reticular activating system (Reprinted from Galambos R (1956). Neural mechanisms of audition. Some recent experiments on the neurophysiology of hearing. Annals of Otology, Rhinology, and Laryngology, *65*, 1055.

function of consciousness. French (1957) considers the reticular activating system to be the principal control center in the central nervous system. This complex neural formation has been pictured as a general alarm mechanism that, upon being activated by incoming neural impulses from sensory stimuli, arouses the cortex so that incoming information can be interpreted.

Figure 14 illustrates the ascending portion of the reticular activating system, which sends projections upward to the surface of various parts of the cerebral cortex, receives input from every sensory modality, and serves an important function in neural integration. The reticular activating system, nestled between the nerve centers of the medulla, extends upward into higher levels of the brainstem and also contains nuclei of the cranial nerves along with nuclei that control such body activity as heart function and respiration (Schnitker, 1972). Nerve fibers from the reticular activating system also descend to the spinal cord to control the sensory stimulation of the spinal cord and the position and tautness of muscles.

Schnitker (1972) also notes that the reticular activating system and the cerebral cortex must receive electrical information in a synchronous manner in order for efficient processing of information to occur. For example, an alert individual's system will receive information via the

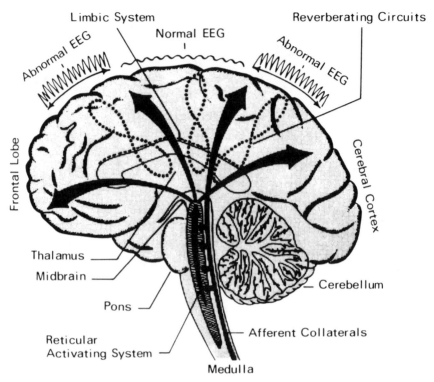

Fig. 14. Reticular activating system (Reprinted from Schnitker M (1972). *The teacher's guide to the brain and learning.* San Rafael, CA: Academic Therapy Publications. p. 14. With permission.)

reticular activating system and the cerebral cortex in time patterns such that the two sources of information will not be in conflict with each other.

The reticular activating system, by virtue of its name, is commonly referred to as the system that "alerts" the brain to new incoming stimuli, but that can also inhibit the function of the brain. Magoun (1963) believes the reticular activating system is discriminative, reasoning that this mechanism assists the cerebral cortex in selecting incoming stimuli that are of paramount importance while inhibiting other stimuli. Ayres (1972) has expanded on this theory by suggesting that children who have a learning disability may have a reticular activating system that fails to discriminate incoming stimuli that should be processed and sent to the cerebral cortex from those that should be suppressed. Therefore, the child is excessively stimulated by having too many sensory signals reaching the cortex and overloading the system. Such overloading would, in essence, preclude discrimination of sensory stimuli that transmit important information for the comprehension of a recent auditory experience. Conversely, we could also postulate that a defective reticular activating system would not carry out its brain-alerting process, thereby preventing important auditory information from being processed adequately by the cortex, since the unalerted cortex would not be properly prepared to process new incoming stimuli.

Another theory concerning faulty auditory processing is that the reticular activating system itself alters the incoming signals from various sensory modalities. If true, a malfunctioning reticular activating system would alter competing sensory information and adversely affect a child's behavior. We have observed in some children that their ability to attend to specific stimuli is disrupted by constantly varying signals in their environment. Such distractions interfere with their ability to perceive and, consequently, learn. From observation, it appears that their central nervous systems are temporarily immobilized by the deluge of incoming stimuli. These children appear to be able to function efficiently only when sensory stimuli are controlled and introduced to the central nervous system in an orderly fashion. Since the reticular activating system serves as a coordinating station for many sensory stimuli, other stimuli such as visual and somatosensory experiences may disrupt the integration process. Therefore, not only can auditory stimuli interfere with processing, but stimuli from other modalities may also inhibit the operation of the reticular activating system.

Goldstein (1967) has theorized that the reticular activating system is not primarily a cortical alerting system; instead, that function is assigned to the lateral lemniscus. He theorizes that the reticular activating system is important in a discriminatory process by which the efferent tracts of the cerebral cortex travel through the reticular activating system carrying autocorrective and integrative information. Carpenter (1972) reports that bilateral lesions of the lateral lemniscus create an EEG wave form similar to that of an animal in a wakeful state. However, lesions of the reticular activating system render wave forms similar to that of an animal in a sleep state. Perhaps, if the lateral lemniscus is not intact, incoming stimuli are transmitted to the cerebral cortex without the benefit of the reticular activating system sorting and suppressing unimportant stimuli. Conversely, if the reticular activating system is not functioning properly, the incoming stimuli are not transmitted efficiently because the reticular activating system is not effectively alerting the cerebral cortex to the arrival of important signals.

Auditory Cortex

The ascending auditory system is completed with the projection of fibers from the medial geniculate body to a region of transverse gyri in the

temporal lobes of the cortex. They fan out in the auditory radiation area
and terminate in the locus of Heschl's gyrus on the floor of the Sylvian
fissure. The latter is illustrated in Figure 15. A series of experiments on
this system, beginning with Campbell's classical work in 1905, have been
conducted in laboratories around the world and continue at the present
time. The results of these efforts, reviewed in great detail by Whitfield
(1967) and more recently by Brugge (1975), have provided a substantial
body of knowledge regarding tonotopical organization and specialized
functions of the auditory cortex, which can be summarized as follows:

1. Each hemisphere receives projections from both ears, so that binaural
    representation of auditory stimuli is present in each temporal lobe.

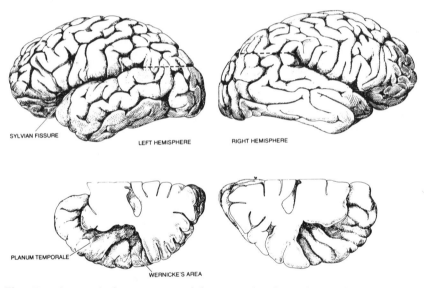

Fig. 15. Anatomical asymmetry of the cortex has been detected in the human
brain and may be related to the distinctive functional specializations of the two
hemispheres. One asymmetry is readily observed in the intact brain: the sylvian
fissure, which defines the upper margin of the temporal lobe, rises more steeply
on the right side of the brain. A more striking asymmetry is found on the planum
temporale, which forms the upper surface of the temporal lobe, and which can be
seen only when the sylvian fissure is opened. The posterior part of the planum
temporale is usually much larger on the left side. The enlarged region is part of
Wernicke's area, suggesting that the asymmetry may be related to the linguistic
dominance of the left hemisphere. The distribution of the asymmetries varies
with handedness (Reprinted from Geschwind N (1979). Specializations of the
human brain. *Scientific American, 241*, 192. With permission.)

2. Each hemisphere maintains the tonotopic organization of the cochlea and brainstem mechanisms by orderly termination of neurons in the auditory radiation area of the cortex.
3. Each hemisphere possesses a "primary" area, which receives fibers from the lower auditory centers, and second- and third-order association areas that surround the primary area and serve elaborating functions.

Unfortunately, as Stillman (1980) has noted, the study of the higher levels of the auditory pathway is complicated since (1) most cells respond poorly in anesthetized animals, and (2) single-cell responses may be poor even in alert-behaving organisms unless the stimulus is of significance to the animal under study. It is obvious, also, that higher-level auditory functions in the human cortex may well be vastly different from those of animals. Nonetheless, anatomical knowledge of the type mentioned serves to remind us of the complex nature of the auditory system and its behavior. An additional factor that lends complexity to the study of the CANS is the progressive rise in cell counts as a function of ascending levels of the system. Chow (1951) estimates the following cell counts for the various levels of the CANS of the monkey:

Cochlear nucleus = 8,800
Superior olivary complex = 34,000
Nucleus of lateral lemniscus = 38,000
Inferior colliculus = 392,000
Mediate geniculate body = 364,000
Auditory cortex = 10,000,000

While difficult to study in spite of highly improved contemporary techniques, studies support the existence of neurons that respond in a variety of ways: (1) those that respond at intervals to periodic sinusoidal changes more predictably than to steady tones; (2) some that respond to frequency changes and not at all to steady tones; (3) those having response areas for frequency-modulated tones that are wider than those mapped for steady tones; (4) neurons that only respond directionally to either rising or falling frequencies; (5) others that exhibit a wide variety of discharge patterns in the same animal call even when the activities of the neurons are recorded within the same vicinity of one another, and (6) still other cells that show the same response to vocalization having widely varying spectra and temporal patterns (Brugge, 1975). There is wide agreement among those doing anatomical and physiological research in audition that stimuli such as pure tones offer little insight into higher-level auditory functions. Perhaps for reasons implicit here, clinicians have turned their attention to tests of CANS-behavior relationships in an effort to define cortical dysfunctions and their behavioral implications. These efforts, which will be considered in Chapter 5, have focused on demonstrating the specialized functions of the two hemispheres. Commenting on hemispheric asymmetry and specialization, Ferry, Culbertson, Fitzgibbons, and Netsky (1979) summarized the current state of knowledge as follows:

> In gross anatomic appearance, the left and right halves of the brain are not identical. The left sylvian fissure is significantly longer than the right in most adult and infant human brains. . . . The superior surface of the posterior temporal lobe is longer on the left. The angular gyrus is smaller on the left. The left planum temporale, the portion of the temporal lobe involved in language comprehension, is distinctly larger than the right. This asymmetry is clearly evident at birth as well as in fetuses as early as 29 weeks gestation, and suggests that the substrate for language development is present well before birth. . . .

This difference in hemisphere structure was illustrated previously in Figure 15. These authors cite Witelson's (1977) evidence of hemispheric specialization: (1) the left hemisphere processes stimuli in a linguistic, sequential, analytic manner to form the basis of receptive and expressive language, and (2) the right hemisphere uses a synthetic or holistic approach. They summarize the differences of the two sides of the brain with the conclusions that the left hemisphere serves language, reading, and mathematical skills, whereas the right hemisphere serves visual-spatial, musical, and mechanical abilities to a greater degree. They also note that boys appear to be more vulnerable than girls to early insult, a fact that they believe may help to explain the higher incidence of language and learning disabilities among boys (Ferry et al, 1979).

Intracortical Connections

While the previously described connections between the brainstem and the cortex are substantial in nature and have been repeatedly confirmed and elaborated, projections among the various areas of the cortex remain relatively vague by comparison. Geschwind (1968) has noted that knowledge is limited because of the questionable transfer of animal research to man and because neuroanatomists have tended to show little interest in cortico-cortical connections. Interest in aphasia has led to the realization that there is neural communication between Wernicke's and Broca's areas via the arcuate fasciculus. The latter, as shown in Figure 16, also has connections with the superior longitudinal fasciculus, thereby facilitating interaction between the visual areas and the angular gyrus, and consequently with the motor areas. However, detailed knowledge of how these diverse areas function within a given hemisphere awaits further research. For example, it is not known why certain children with

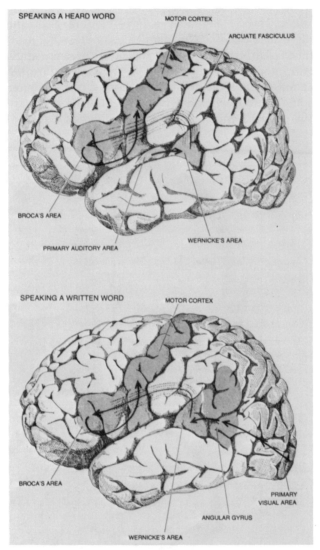

Fig. 16. Intracortical connections via the arcuate fasciculus. Linguistic competence requires the cooperation of several areas of the cortex. When a word is heard (upper diagram), the sensation from the ears is received by the primary auditory cortex, but the word cannot be understood until the signal has been processed in Wernicke's area nearby. If the word is to be spoken, some representation of it is thought to be transmitted from Wernicke's area to Broca's area, through a bundle of nerve fibers called the arcuate fasciculus. In Broca's area the word evokes a detailed program for articulation, which is supplied to the face area of the motor cortex. The motor cortex in turn drives the muscles of the lips, the tongue, the larynx, and so on (Reprinted from Geschwind N (1979). Specializations of the human brain. *Scientific American, 241,* 190. With permission.)

central auditory processing deficits have reading difficulties, or vice versa, while others do not. However, the commissural system, which serves as the final link that completes the auditory chain, appears to offer an important information source. As illustrated in Figure 17, the *corpus callosum* is a massive bundle of fibers that connects the two hemispheres, thus providing communication between the functional processes of each (perhaps the proper term is "both"). Gazzaniga and LeDoux (1978) pre-

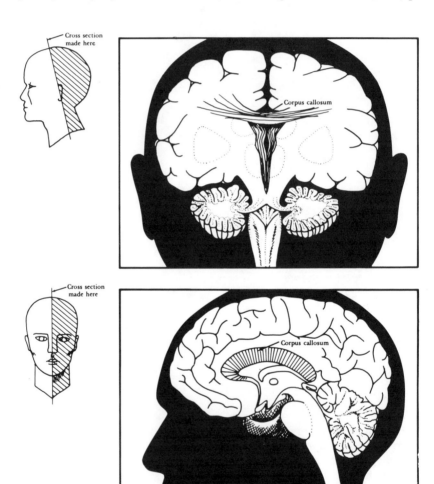

Fig. 17. Two views of the cerebral hemispheres and the corpus callosum, the major nerve-fiber tract connecting them (Reprinted from Lindsay P, & Norman D (1972). Human information processing. New York: Academic Press, p. 315. With permission.)

sent an intriguing treatment of the two hemispheres, the specialization found in each, and their cooperative nature via the corpus collosum. They are persuaded, based on their direct assessment of a series of "split-brain" patients made available to them by Dartmouth Medical School, that dual cerebral hemispheres subserve sensorimotor rather than cognitive functions, since it is only the former that suffer following hemispherectomy. They also stress the importance of the transfer of function between hemispheres, which work in intimately associated synchrony. While most of these authors' attention is directed to visual and manual behaviors, subsequent work on auditory factors at Dartmouth has confirmed parallel behaviors with audition (Musiek, Pinheiro, & Wilson, 1980; Musiek, Wilson, & Reeves, 1981).

The CANS, of course, also has a descending system by which the complex neural events that culminate at the cortical level transmit response information to the various stations of the brainstem, and, to some degree, even to the cochlea. The descending (efferent) system apparently provides further refinement to the total process, which is still poorly understood except for the inhibitory action it communicates to the hair cells (Rasmussen, 1960). Nauta and Feirtag (1979) remind us that the central nervous system consists of billions of neurons and that a single neuron may connect with thousands of others. They constitute a computational network, the complexity and enormity of which is incredible. However, it seems to us that only through expanding our knowledge of this marvelous system can we begin to understand its behavioral correlates of auditory, visual, language, and learning processes. For the reader who wishes to pursue this subject in greater depth than is possible here, we recommend two excellent sources: Springer and Deutsch (1981) and Kinsbourne (1978).

3

Behavior Manifestations

For the past decade or so, parents, teachers, psychologists, other school personnel, and children with known central auditory problems have assisted us in developing a profile of behaviors that are characteristic of children with CAPD. Hopefully, this profile will aid audiologists, parents, and school personnel in developing an awareness of those clues that signal when a child should be "red flagged" for an evaluation for CAPD. Conditions such as peripheral hearing loss, speech and language problems, and visual acuity dysfunction are often initially suspected on the basis of atypical behaviors that the child demonstrates. Similarly, we need to define those characteristics that are common attributes of children with central auditory problems. Hopefully, a good screening test can be developed in the future for initial identification; at present, however, we must rely upon recognition of the behavioral traits associated with CAPD. The major problem areas that continue to surface in case histories include: (1) auditory behaviors, (2) intellectual function and academic achievement, (3) physical considerations, (4) speech and language skills, and (5) social behaviors. A discussion of each area is presented to aid clinicians in exploring possible clues for initially referring a child for a central auditory processing problem.

AUDITORY BEHAVIORS

The child with CAPD frequently evidences inconsistent awareness of sound; he is not always alerted by new auditory stimuli in the way that normal children are. He may be classified as a "poor listener" because of his tendency to ignore certain auditory stimuli. He may say "Huh?" or "What?" frequently, behaving as a hearing-impaired child who needs to have auditory input repeated. Conversely, the CAPD child is often easily distracted at home or in the classroom. He may also have a very short auditory attention span and appear to be unable to attend to a given task for any length of time. He constantly appears unable to sustain attention to a particular task. He may evidence slow or delayed responses to verbal stimuli; the child may need to "buy time" in order to process auditory information adequately. We believe that many of his perceived messages are sufficiently degraded so that he needs more time to integrate them. The CAPD child may also have difficulty with phonics, especially when phonic drills are conducted in noisy or distracting environments. While not all CAPD children have phonic difficulties, they do have poorer auditory discrimination for social discourse in noisy listening environments than when the environment is quiet. That is, although some children are adequate listeners in favorable circumstances, their comprehension breaks down in the presence of competing stimuli for reasons that are apparently unrelated to phonics skills. This problem is illustrated when they continue to look quizzically at the teacher or parent as though they heard the message but failed to *understand* what was said to them. In other words, they simply have trouble following verbal instructions or questions, and the problem is exaggerated under unfavorable listening conditions.

INTELLECTUAL FUNCTION AND
ACADEMIC ACHIEVEMENT

Many professionals have asked if intellectual capacity can be used as an indicator of a CAPD. Is intelligence a factor that can help us to determine if a child has an auditory learning disability? A given child's intellectual capability is important when it is viewed in the light of his academic achievement. The intellectual quotient is not necessarily important in itself, but it can provide diagnostic insight when it fails to correlate with classroom proficiency. Specifically, children with CAPD typically have lower academic achievement than would be expected from their IQs. This relationship often comes as a surprise to teachers and parents, but it can serve as a basis for referral for evaluation for learning problems, including CAPD. The CAPD children we have seen clinically over the past ten years have exhibited intelligence levels from low-normal to genius, and, regardless of their intellectual skills, their performance in school is inordinately poor. This discrepancy between potential and performance is perplexing for both parents and teachers and probably for the child. The children are usually bewildered and frustrated by their inability to succeed in school.

Many referrals for a central auditory evaluation have come from psychologists who noticed that a child's performance on the Wechsler Intelligence Scale for Children (WISC) or other intelligence tests did not compare favorably with the child's performance on measures such as the

Wide Range Achievement Test (WRAT).

Some psychologists have speculated that children who have an auditory perceptual dysfunction will routinely have lower scores on the verbal subtests of the WISC than they will on the performance subtests of the same measure. They reason that a child with a CAPD will be deficient in verbal skills because of their belief in the theoretical relationship between audition and language. It is also assumed that such children will rely more heavily on visual skills. Although the latter may be true, it remains to be supported by data. Nonetheless, we have not seen a predictable relationship between children's results on WISC subtests and CAPD. For example, some children with a confirmed CAPD receive better scores on verbal subtests of the WISC while others receive better scores on the performance subtests. Therefore, reliance on the relationship between verbal and performance subtests cannot serve in lieu of auditory tests and does not seem to be diagnostically helpful in initially identifying a child with a CAPD. However, it remains to be seen how those subtests might relate to linguistic versus nonlinguistic central auditory tests. Table 5, which illustrates this point, presents WISC scores supplied from referral source psychological records on 35 randomly selected children with confirmed CAPD who were evaluated at our clinic. While 22 subjects did indeed have higher scores on the performance scale, 13 had higher verbal-scale scores. This result would seem to support our contention that WISC verbal-subtest scores are not a valid predictor of central auditory integrity.

PHYSICAL CONSIDERATIONS

With rare exceptions, children with CAPD do not exhibit an observable physical health problem. Both general medical and neurological examinations are typically unremarkable. An occasional child with a CAPD may exhibit a mildly abnormal EEG, but the vast majority of children who have been referred for both general physical and neurological evaluations show negative results, including EEG findings.

Schoenfeld (1975) has also observed negative EEG profiles in children with confirmed CAPD. Apparently, CAPDs in children are sufficiently subtle that they elude identification by EEG. It may also be that,

Table 5
Summary of WISC Scale Raw Scores for 35 Randomly
Selected Children with Confirmed CAPD

Higher Performance than Verbal Scores:	22
Higher Verbal than Performance Scores:	13*

*Some differences were small, but ranged from 7 to 28 points on 7 of the 13 subjects.

since EEG measures cortical function, subcortical involvements would naturally preclude detection by this method.

It should be noted that if a child complains of severe headaches, dizziness, blackouts, hearing problems, visual difficulties, and/or unexplained motor difficulties, a neurological referral should be made immediately. These symptoms can occur in any combination and may signal the presence of a space-occupying lesion. Thorough central auditory evaluation by the audiologist can also aid the neurologist in identifying the presence and location of the problem.

SPEECH AND LANGUAGE SKILLS

It is now clear that children with CAPD do not necessarily manifest language or speech problems (Ludlow, 1980; Tallal & Newcombe, 1978; Thal & Barone, 1983; Willeford & Billger, 1978). In our experience, some children do have language and/or speech difficulties, but many of the children we evaluate do not. It is possible, of course, that undetected subtle speech-language dysfunctions may have been present at a very early age in the children in our population.

Some youngsters in our population have had very mild articulation errors, fluency problems, and/or mild word-order problems. Others have manifested moderate-to-severe language delays that, of course, may invalidate certain test results. If a child does have a significant language delay, the language age of the child is very important when selecting appropriate CAP tests.

It can be theorized that a child with a CAPD should have a speech and language problem as a result of that deficiency. Although this theory has merit, CAPDs of the type we see in children are manifested primarily when a child is in difficult listening environments. During the early speech and language years, the child is in the favorable auditory environment of the home and experiences little auditory confusion as he is learning to use language and developing articulation skills. Therefore, a child with a CAPD will not necessarily manifest a noticeable speech and/or language abnormality. However, when the child starts school or enters other environments that tax his auditory system to a greater degree, he begins to experience difficulty understanding verbal messages. That appears to be the sequence of events that leads to social and academic problems in the absence of speech or language disorders.

SOCIAL BEHAVIORS

Apart from academic, auditory, medical, and speech-language manifestations, children with CAPD also exhibit social behaviors that are atypical in nature. Many such children are described as hyperactive or as exhibiting a high activity level. Some of them are given drugs, such as ritalin, in an attempt to reduce their levels of activity. Many of these children are labeled as "behavior problems" both at home and at school. It is tempting to hypothesize that these children are having trouble coping with their auditory world. They act out in confusion and frustration, and increased activity levels result. In some, their emotional state may combine with subtle organic disturbances to produce hyperactivity. The increased activity levels in some children may result from their need to use much more energy than average children in order to pay attention and understand what is being taught in school. They have to work harder to sort out crucial auditory information and go through superfluous motion in the process. Lehmann, Creswell, and Huffman (1965) have shown that greater energy is expended by normal subjects when performing tasks in the presence of noise. Downs and Crum (1978) found similar results and predicted that learning-disabled children would likely show even greater energy expenditure in their efforts to interact with their environments.

Other children with CAPD exhibit *lower* than normal activity levels. They do not act up in the classroom; on the contrary, they appear lethargic, passive, reserved, or fatigued. Parents report that they seem "worn out" after school.

Teachers frequently describe children with CAPD as "slow starters" and complain that they fail to complete assigned tasks. Such behaviors are not surprising if the child has failed to understand the teacher's instructions, and Toman (1969) reports that 70 percent of the talking in classrooms is done by teachers. Thus, children must depend heavily on accurate auditory input. Perhaps this is also why they seem to have apparent memory problems and difficulty organizing information. Both of these behaviors are natural consequences of "not having understood" the teacher's verbal instructions. Our experience is that there is a fine line between distorted auditory input that leaves the child little to remember and a true memory problem. We believe many children with CAPD have been mislabeled as having poor memory. For example, several children in our client population have shown excellent memory in the protected environment of our clinic, even though they are undergoing memory training elsewhere. Moreover, Gallagher, Toby, Cullen, and Rampp (1976), on the basis of experiments to compare memory functions of CAPD children and a group of matched normals, concluded that those with CAPD have difficulty in initial input and processing of acoustic input rather than in retrieval of signal information.

Many parents describe their CAPD child as a daydreamer, which also seems an expected behavior if the child is a poor listener or doesn't understand faint, distorted, or complex messages. If their auditory world is confusing and unrewarding, it seems reasonable that they would withdraw into the security of daydreams.

OTHER BEHAVIORS

Other behaviors that are manifested by children with CAPD include disruptive classroom pranks, asocial behaviors ranging from withdrawal to hostile aggressiveness, delinquency, and even suicidal fantasies (Meyer, 1975). A considerable number of the children we see are referred from the local mental health clinic or from private-practice psychologists who are seeing the children for behavior management therapy.

Quite a number of CAPD children tend to be "loners," preferring to play by themselves. Others have a tendency to prefer the company of younger children or to be around adults rather than with companions of their own age. We suspect that this selective choice of friends and associates may be the way in which the child controls his auditory world in order to find social acceptance. The child does not have to compete as much as he does with children his own age. Parents often tell us that the child does not like to be with children his own age, especially during play activities or in confusing listening environments such as the school lunchroom. Remembering these situations in our own childhood helps us to appreciate the pressures of trying to fit in with the crowd and trying to participate in games, conversations, or other peer-related activities. We can understand why participation in group activities may increase anxiety on the part of the child with a CAPD.

It should be emphasized that not all of these children will experience all of these difficulties in their everyday environments. Moreover, we cannot attribute all atypical behavior a child may demonstrate to his auditory deficiencies. Some children with confirmed CAPD will be so overwhelmed by their inability to function adequately that they become devastated by their environment. Others will experience some frustrations during their daily tasks, but they handle them with minimal adversity. In our experience, some children have experienced such frequent failure during their life that they are literally in a failure cycle and tend to "give up." In retrospect, some parents believe they could have anticipated their child's impending academic and social difficulties on the basis of the child's clinging behavior in active, congested environments that were exciting and fun for the siblings. The parents disclaim fear as the basis for this behavior, feeling, rather, that the child was simply overwhelmed by the situations. Other parents tell us their children seek the solace and quiet security of their rooms after school. They like to be read to or have discussions in that atmosphere. A few even retire to their rooms and play loud music, which is seen as a way of stabilizing a normally dynamic and difficult auditory world.

The guidelines for initial referral for a central auditory processing evaluation are basically behavioral in nature. A screening test that is sensitive enough to identify most CAPD children reliably has not been developed at this time. However, if teachers, parents, and pediatricians keep the common manifestations in mind, appropriate referrals and early identification can be made.

Fisher (1976) has developed a checklist to help identify children who may have a central auditory dysfunction. It can be used by teachers or other school personnel to help classify academic performance and related behaviors that make children suspect for a CAPD. This checklist is used in a number of school settings for this purpose, but some school audiologists feel that it yields a high false-positive rate for early identification of children with potential problems. Another checklist, developed by Willeford and Burleigh for use in a research project, involves a rating scale by which behaviors associated with CAPD can be numerically ranked. This checklist has not been utilized widely, and its sensitivity, reliability, and validity remain to be shown. However, both of these checklists may prove to be increasingly useful with CAPD children, including those who are too severely involved to perform more formal diagnostic tests. The checklists are shown in Figures 18 and 19, and the behaviors discussed in this section are summarized in Table 6.

Table 6
Common Behaviors of Children with Central
Auditory Disorders

Poor listener
Poor attention (short span)
Easily distracted
Misunderstands
Trouble following verbal instructions
Frustration
Poor speech discrimination
Poor ability to organize information
Seemingly has poor memory
Slow starter
Doesn't complete tasks
Daydreams
Hyperactive or hypoactive
Hostility
Disruptive
Withdrawal
A "loner"—often plays by self
Prefers company of "younger" friends or adults
"Soft," if any, neurological signs
"Clings" to parents (young child) in active environments
Seeks quiet or structured environment

Student's Name _____ District/Building _____

Date _____ Grade _____ Observer _____ Position _____

Please place a check mark before each item that is considered to be a concern by the observer.

_____1. History of hearing loss.

_____2. History of ear infection(s).

_____3. Does not pay attention (listen) to instruction 50% or more of the time.

_____4. Does not listen carefully to directions—often necessary to repeat instructions.

_____5. Says "Huh?" or "What?" at least five or more times per day.

_____6. Student cannot attend to auditory stimuli for more than a few seconds.

_____7. Short attention span. (If item is checked, also check the most appropriate time frame.)
     _____0–2 minutes   _____ 5–15 minutes

     _____2–5 minutes   _____15–30 minutes

_____8. Daydreams—attention drifts—not with it at times.

_____9. Easily distracted by background sound(s).

_____10. Difficulty with phonics.

_____11. Problems with sound discrimination.

_____12. Trouble recalling a sequence student has heard.

_____13. Forgets what is said in a few minutes.

_____14. Does not remember simple routine things from day to day.

_____15. Problems recalling what was heard last week, month, year.

_____16. Difficulty following auditory directions.

_____17. Often misunderstands what is said.

_____18. Does not comprehend many words—verbal concepts for age/grade level.

_____19. Slow or delayed response to verbal stimuli.

_____20. Has a language problem (morphology, syntax, vocabulary, phonology).

_____21. Has an articulation (phonology) problem.

_____22. Child cannot always relate what is heard with what is seen.

_____23. Learns poorly through the auditory channel.

_____24. Lacks motivation to learn.

_____25. Performance is below average in one or more subject area(s).

Scoring: Four percent credit for each numbered item *not* checked.

Number of items *not* checked _____ × 4 = _____.

Fig. 18 Fisher's Auditory Problems Checklist. (Reprinted from Fisher L. (1976). *Fisher's Auditory Problems Checklist*, Bemidji, Mn: Life Products. With permission.)

On a scale of 1 (never) to 5 (always), rate the student's ability on the following:

	Never	Occasion-ally	Often	Usually	Always
1. Has difficulty in paying attention to speaker	1	2	3	4	5
2. Is a poor listener	1	2	3	4	5
3. Disturbed by background sound/noise:					
SPECIFICALLY:					
a. speech	1	2	3	4	5
b. whispering	1	2	3	4	5
c. shuffling papers, feet, etc.	1	2	3	4	5
d. pencil sharpener	1	2	3	4	5
e. playground noise	1	2	3	4	5
f. from other classrooms or halls	1	2	3	4	5
g. other (class bells, etc.)	1	2	3	4	5
_____					
4. Daydreams	1	2	3	4	5
5. Has short attention span	1	2	3	4	5
6. Misunderstands verbal instructions	1	2	3	4	5
7. Misunderstands written instructions	1	2	3	4	5
8. Asks to repeat verbal instructions	1	2	3	4	5
9. Slow or delayed response to verbal stimuli	1	2	3	4	5
10. Has trouble recalling verbal material originally understood	1	2	3	4	5

1. Decreased performance in
   the following subjects:

Mathematics	1	2	3	4	5
Reading	1	2	3	4	5
Spelling	1	2	3	4	5
Phonics	1	2	3	4	5
Language Arts	1	2	3	4	5
Other _____	1	2	3	4	5

2. Slow starter   1   2   3   4   5
3. Difficulty completing tasks 1   2   3   4   5
4. Child relies heavily on   1   2   3   4   5
   visual clues in classroom
5. Receives resource-tutorial
   help
   (Type) _____
6. Receives speech/language   1   2   3   4   5
   therapy

1. Impulsive   1   2   3   4   5
2. Frustrated   1   2   3   4   5
3. Withdrawn   1   2   3   4   5
4. Aggressive   1   2   3   4   5
5. Not accepted by peers   1   2   3   4   5
6. Prefers association   1   2   3   4   5
   with younger children
7. Child is a "loner"   1   2   3   4   5
8. Restless/excessive   1   2   3   4   5
   physical movement
9. Disturbs other children   1   2   3   4   5
   during class
10. Gives up easily   1   2   3   4   5
11. Seeks assistance   1   2   3   4   5
    from teacher
12. Insensitive to time   1   2   3   4   5
    responsibilities

Fig. 19.   Willeford and Burleigh Behavior Rating Scale for Central Auditory
Disorders

Case History

Obtaining comprehensive case history information is a vital part of every audiological evaluation, and this is especially true when evaluating the child with a suspected central auditory processing dysfunction. The audiologist has a special responsibility for gathering historical information that will offer direction in evaluating and managing a child's ability to process auditory information. Indeed, a thorough and appropriate case history, in our judgment, provides the very foundation for diagnosis and treatment.

Ehrlich (1978) believes that a good case history serves three important functions. First, the case history seeks information from the child's parents, a process that helps to get the parents actively involved in the evaluation process. This gives them an opportunity to express their concerns about their child's health, behavior, educational achievement, and interpersonal relationships, which is invaluable information to the diagnostician and is extremely important in directing the clinician toward the child's needs.

Second, Ehrlich maintains that the case history can help the examiner to identify the parents' current concerns and, at the same time, aid in the selection of appropriate tests for the evaluation. We feel that information such as the child's reading ability, language level, and an overall behavior profile can provide the clinician with insights that will help to determine the appropriate directions to follow when administering and interpreting diagnostic tests.

Third, Ehrlich points out that the case history will, hopefully, provide information that can support or challenge test results that are obtained. We agree that the use of a cross-check is important when evaluating any child, and the case history can serve as a guide by which test findings can be supported. However, the precision of such cross-checks depends on good clinical judgment.

There are other important reasons why gathering information from a child's parents in the form of a case history can be helpful. Since the study of CAPD is relatively new, and the causes are largely speculative, information gleaned from case histories can provide valuable insights about the possible causes of central auditory dysfunctions. The suggested causes of CAPD are numerous and quite varied. The relationship between adults with CANS insult and central auditory disorders is well documented (Berlin & Lowe, 1972; Bocca & Calearo, 1963; Jerger, 1960, 1964; Jerger & Jerger, 1975a, 1975b; Katz, 1968; Katz & Pack, 1975; Kimura, 1961; Lynn & Gilroy, 1975, 1977; Milner, 1962; Speaks, 1975), but the direct transfer of that relationship to children with CAPD is complicated by a number of factors: (1) the CAPD child generally reveals only soft neurological signs (see Table 7), if any; (2) the child is still undergoing physiological and perceptual maturation, and (3) children are more vulnerable to environmental and cultural influences. Thus, neuropsychological functions in children require further research to confirm and clarify these relationships.

Many of the purported causes of learning disabilities (LD) and CAPD have medical orientations that, interestingly, are often ignored in the psychoeducational literature. The latter frequently deals only with the symptomatic characteristics. It should also be kept in mind that potential causes may occur singly or may coexist with one or more of the others.

Table 7
Borderline, Equivocal, or "Soft" Neurological Signs
in Children

Clumsiness in tasks requiring fine motor coordination (tying shoelaces or
    doing buttons)
Choreiform movements
Mild dysphasia
Associated movements
Borderline hyperreflexia and reflex asymmetries
Finger agnosia
Dysdiadochokinesis
Ocular apraxia and endpoint nystagmus
Tremor
Graphesthesias
Whirling
Extinction to double simultaneous tactile stimulation
Pupillary inequalities
Mixed laterality and disturbances of right-left discrimination
Unilateral winking defect
Awkward gait
Avoiding response in outstretched hands

From Schain R. *Neurology of childhood learning disorders* (ed 2). Baltimore: Williams &
Wilkins, 1977. With permission.

Obviously, since little hard data exist on the causes of deficient auditory processing, research is urgently needed. This is particularly true since many of the treatment strategies have an etiological basis.

Case histories can also reveal information relative to the behavior profile of the child. For example, some children exhibit high activity levels, whereas others perform in a lethargic manner. Such behaviors are common concomitants of CAPD. Although abnormal activity levels may be related to other disorders, awareness of these behaviors and their frequent association with CAPD can lead to earlier diagnosis of these children and, hopefully, avoid the school failures and frustrations that become personal traumas.

Finally, case history information can often offer guidance for managing these children. Our clinical experience has taught us a great deal about which environments create difficulties for children with CAPD. Some of that information was gained directly from parent comments during the case history interview. We have become aware of those situations that are most difficult for children with CAPD and, consequently, have devised ways of helping those children learn to cope with adverse listening situations. Both teachers and parents have been valuable sources of guidance for us in this regard by monitoring which types of suggestions were helpful to the children at home and at school. We are confident that continued communication with parents, teachers, and counselors will provide even greater information concerning the management of these children. It is important that clinicians foster a relaxed and open atmosphere during a case history session in order to facilitate the flow of information from the informant.

The format of a case history varies widely from one clinical setting to another. To our knowledge, a model case history for CAPD has not appeared in the literature. For that reason, the reader may find the case histories shown in Figures 20 and 21 of interest. The case history shown in Figure 20 was our primary history form until recently, when it was revised, as shown in Figure 21, so that history information could be easily transferred to a computer program. We are currently in the process of accumulating case history data in an effort to analyze trends regarding such factors as etiologies, family history, and speech and language profiles. These particular histories have been modified periodically as we gained new information about CAPD.

Taking a central auditory case history requires planning since it is important for the clinician to ask questions that range from general to very specific. We mail our case history form to the family and ask them to complete it prior to the child's evaluation. The diagnostician then reviews the completed form with the informant(s) at the time of the evaluation in the event that some entries are not clear or are incomplete. This history

Date:_____ Date Evaluated:_____

Name_____ Age:_____ Date of Birth:_____

Address:_____ Sex: _____

_____

Home telephone:_____ Work telephone:_____

School:_____ Grade:_____ Teachers:_____

Child's physician:_____ City:_____

Who referred your child to this center?_____

Reason for testing?_____

FAMILY BACKGROUND:

Father's name: _____ Age:_____

   Health: Occupation:

_____   _____

Mother's name: _____ Age:_____

   Health: Occupation:

_____   _____

Other children in family:

Name	Age	Sex	Health
_____	____	___	_____
_____	____	___	_____
_____	____	___	_____
_____	____	___	_____
_____	____	___	_____

HEARING & SPEECH INFORMATION:

Has your child had any ear infections, abscesses, drainage, or other ear problems? If so, please name and list: age, how frequent, duration, how resolved.

_____

_____

Fig. 20   Central Auditory Processing Case History

64

Has your child had any treatment for his/her ears? (include tonsillectomy, adenoidectomy, tubes, medication, lancing)

_____

Does any member of the family currently have (or previously had) a suspected hearing problem and/or wear a hearing aid?

_____

Has any family member had an operation for their ears? If so, at what age & date?

_____

Does your child's hearing seem to fluctuate (get better, then poorer)?_____

Has it ever been suggested that your child had a speech problem? If so, did he/she receive speech therapy? (at what age, how long)

_____

Please describe any other examinations, tests, or evaluations that your child has had:

	Where	When	Age	Results
Hearing Evaluations	_____	_____	____	_____
Neurologic (EEG)	_____	_____	____	_____
Psychological Intelligence Tests	_____	_____	____	_____
Speech & Language	_____	_____	____	_____
Vision	_____	_____	____	_____

Other_____

MEDICAL HISTORY—Prenatal:

Did the mother suffer any illnesses or was she exposed to illness?_____

Was the mother involved in any accidents?_____

Did she ever require blood transfusions?_____

Was the mother under any medication? If so, for what, name of medication,

length taken?_____

Was there a problem of blood incompatibility (Rh factor)_____

Did the mother suffer from toxemia?_____

65

Was the mother exposed to alcohol and/or drugs? If so, amount, duration, side effects?_____

Has mother suffered any previous miscarriages?_____

Did mother suffer any undue stress or anxiety?_____

Was mother ever exposed to loud noise levels? If so, duration, side effects?

_____

Was the mother on any special diets (weight gain/loss, low sugar, vegetarian)?

_____

Describe any other problems or concerns you may have had before birth:

_____

_____

MEDICAL HISTORY—Natal

What was the length of pregnancy?_____

What was the length of labor?_____

What was the child's birthweight?_____

Were any anesthetics required? If so, name?_____

Were any instruments used?_____

Was the child a breech birth?_____

Was the child born by Caesarean section (C-section)?_____

Did the child suffer any breathing problems?_____

Was auxiliary breathing apparatus required?_____

Was there any discoloration?_____

Describe any complications or other concerns during birth:_____

_____

_____

MEDICAL HISTORY—Postnatal:

Did your child have any scars, bruises, deformation at birth? Describe.

_____

Fig. 20   Central Auditory Processing Case History (continued)

Did your child have swallowing or sucking problems?_____

Did your child have feeding difficulties?_____

Please list all childhood diseases (including age, duration, severity, treatment, complications):

_____

_____

_____

Does your child have allergies? If so, please list and indicate medication.

_____

Has your child been hospitalized? If so, reason, age, duration, treatment:

_____

Has your child been involved in any accidents (describe)?_____

_____

Has your child suffered any head traumas (age, severity)?_____

Has your child experienced any seizures or convulsions? If so, frequency of occurrence, age, severity, duration, treatment:_____

_____

Has your child experienced recurrent headaches?_____

Has your child suffered from dizziness? (age, severity, treatment)_____

_____

Has your child suffered any complications associated with medical treatment? If so, describe. _____

Please list all medication your child has taken or is currently taking:

Medication	Dosage	Age	Length	Illness
_____	_____	_____	_____	_____
_____	_____	_____	_____	_____
_____	_____	_____	_____	_____

Has your child been placed on any special diets or is he/she currently on a special diet? (include weight gain/loss, low-sodium, vegetarian, low-sugar, etc.)

_____

DEVELOPMENTAL HISTORY:

What hand does your child prefer to use?_____

At what age did this preference appear?_____

Is your child clumsy or accident prone?_____

At what age did your child begin to walk?_____ To talk?_____

Has the child had a recent physical examination? If so, by whom and when:

_____

SOCIAL AND ENVIRONMENTAL INFORMATION:

Do you feel that your child is overly sensitive to loud noise?_____

Does your child appear confused when he is in noisy places?_____

Does your child seem to follow and understand television programs?_____

Has your child ever been exposed to loud noise for short periods of time?____

for longer, more continuous periods of time?_____
(i.e., basketball games, concerts). Please indicate at what age, duration of

exposure, severity:_____

_____

Is your child living in a bilingual environment?_____

If so, what other language is spoken?_____

Does your child, or has your child, preferred to play by himself?_____

Or does he prefer to play with other children?_____

Does your child ask questions or make statements that other people might
consider foolish, irrelevant, or immature?_____

Is your child easily frustrated?_____

Is your child easily distractible?_____

Is your child hyperactive?_____ Underactive?_____

Does your child appear to have a short attention span?_____

Does your child daydream?_____

Is your child forgetful?_____

Does your child lack motivation?_____

Fig. 20 Central Auditory Processing Case History (continued)

Does your child tire easily? If so, under what conditions?_____

Is your child impulsive?_____

Has your child been under any stress, pressure, or anxiety at home or school?_____

Please describe any other problems or concerns you may have observed:___

_____

EDUCATIONAL INFORMATION:

Has your child ever repeated a grade?_____ If so, what grade, reason:

_____

Is your child presently in an open or traditional classroom?_____

Has your child ever been in an open classroom?_____

Has your child ever received special help at school?_____

    If so, please describe:_____

Does your child like school?_____

Please indicate those subjects with which your child has the most difficulty:

_____

What subjects does your child excel in?_____

What are his favorite subjects?_____

Has your child had behavioral problems at school? If so, describe:

_____

Have any relatives had difficulty learning to read or had other learning problems in school (include parents, siblings, grandparents, etc.)? If so, describe.

_____

Have any teachers ever asked you to have your child's hearing tested?_____

    Or vision tested?_____

Does your child appear to rely more heavily on visual cues in the classroom?

_____

Has your child ever used earmuffs or earplugs at school?_____

At home?_____

    Or under special conditions? (please specify)_____

Does your child have problems following directions?_____

Has your child been involved with alcohol and/or drugs? If so, please describe:

_____

Has your child ever had difficulty with the law? If so, please describe:

_____

Please describe any further information about your child's behavior, health, schooling, etc., which you feel is important.

_____

_____

_____

_____

THANK YOU FOR YOUR COOPERATION.

Fig. 20   Central Auditory Processing Case History

Case Number:_____ Audiologist_____

Date_____ Date Evaluated_____

Name_____ Age_____ Date of Birth_____

Address_____

City_____ State_____ Sex_____M_____F

Home Telephone_____ Work Telephone_____

School_____ Grade_____ Teacher_____

Child's Physician_____ City_____

Who referred your child to this center? _____Audiologist

_____Neurologist

_____Other Physicians

_____Private Psychologist

_____School Personnel

_____Speech & Language Pathologist

_____Agencies

_____Self Referred

Reason for testing? _____Academic Difficulties

_____Speech and Language Problems

_____Emotional Problems

_____Reading Problems

_____Hearing Disorder

Family Background

Father's Name_____ Age_____

Health: _____Excellent _____Good _____Adequate _____Poor

If adequate or poor, what is/are the reason(s):_____

_____

_____

Fig. 21 Central Auditory Disorder Case History

Mother's Name _____ Age _____

    Health: _____Excellent _____Good _____Adequate _____Poor

    If adequate or poor, what is/are the reason(s): _____

_____

_____

Other Children in Family:

Name	Age	(M or F)	Good Listener
_____	_____	_____	____Yes ____No
_____	_____	_____	____Yes ____No
_____	_____	_____	____Yes ____No
_____	_____	_____	____Yes ____No
_____	_____	_____	____Yes ____No
_____	_____	_____	____Yes ____No

Hearing and Speech Information

	Age	# Episodes	Duration
Ear Infections	_____	_____	____weeks ____months
Abscesses	_____	_____	____weeks ____months
Drainage	_____	_____	____weeks ____months
Other	_____	_____	____weeks ____months

Has your child had any treatment for his/her ears? ____Yes ____No

If yes, type: ____Tonsillectomy

             ____Adenoidectomy

             ____Tubes

             ____Medication

             ____Lancing

             ____Other

Does any member of the family currently have (or previously had) a *suspected*

hearing problem? ____Yes ____No If so, family member(s) _____

_____

_____

Fig. 21   Central Auditory Disorder Case History (continued)

Does any member of the family currently wear a hearing aid? ___Yes ___No

If yes, relationship_____

Has any member of the family had an operation involving their ears?
___Yes ___No

If yes,

Type	Age	Results Good	No Change
Mastoiditis	_____	_____	_____
Stapedectomy	_____	_____	_____
Myringotomy (tubes)	_____	_____	_____
Tympanoplasty	_____	_____	_____
Other	_____	_____	_____

Does your child's hearing seem to fluctuate (get better, then poorer)?
___Yes ___No

Has it ever been suggested that your child has a speech or language problem?

___Yes ___No   If yes,   Type   Age Diagnosed

Type	Age Diagnosed
Articulation	_____
Language	_____
Stuttering	_____
Auditory Perception	_____
Voice Disorders	_____
Aphasia	_____
Other_____	_____

Maternal History

Did mother suffer (or was she exposed to) any of the following during pregnancy?

	Yes	No	Month of Pregnancy
German Measles (Rubella)----	_____	_____	_____
Other Virus (list)_____	_____	_____	_____
Influenza	_____	_____	_____
Chicken Pox	_____	_____	_____
Mumps ---------------------------	_____	_____	_____

73

Toxemia   _____ _____ _____

Bleeding   _____ _____ _____

Threatened Abortion   _____ _____ _____

Diabetes   _____ _____ _____

Maternal Syphilis--------------- _____ _____ _____

Radiation   _____ _____ _____ If yes, amount_____

Maternal Malnutrition   _____ _____ _____

Maternal Anemia   _____ _____ _____

Alcoholism   _____ _____ _____

Drug Addiction ----------------- _____ _____ _____ If yes, type_____

Immunizations   _____ _____ _____ If yes, type_____

Smoking   _____ _____ _____

Caffeine (all sources)   _____ _____ _____

Accidents   _____ _____ _____ If yes, type_____

Blood Transfusions ------------- _____ _____ _____

Medication   _____ _____ _____ If yes, type_____

Rh Incompatibility   _____ _____ _____

Miscarriages   _____ _____ _____

Special Diets   _____ _____ _____ If yes, type_____

Exposed to loud noise -------- _____ _____ _____ If yes, amount_____

Undue stress & anxiety   _____ _____ _____

Other concerns or problems   _____ _____ _____

     during pregnancy   _____

Birth History

Length of pregnancy? ___5 mo. ___6 mo. ___7 mo. ___8 mo.
___9 mo. ___10 mo. _____Other

Length of labor? _____hours ____days

Child's birthweight: _____Less than 4 lbs. ___4–10 lbs. ___11 lbs. over

Fig. 21 Central Auditory Disorder Case History (continued)

Were the following conditions associated with the birth of your child?

	Yes	No
Instruments Used (forceps, etc.)	_____	_____
Breech Birth	_____	_____
Caesarean	_____	_____
Breathing Problems	_____	_____
Breathing Apparatus Required	_____	_____
Discoloration	_____	_____

Natal History

Did your child suffer any of the following after birth?

	Yes	No
Scars	_____	_____
Bruises	_____	_____
Deformation (if yes, type)_____	_____	_____
Feeding Difficulties	_____	_____
Swallowing Problems	_____	_____
Sucking Problems	_____	_____

Postnatal History

Has your child had the following? If yes, note severity:

	Yes	No	Mild	Severity Mod.	Severe
Measles (Red)	_____	_____	_____	_____	_____
Mumps	_____	_____	_____	_____	_____
Measles (German)	_____	_____	_____	_____	_____
Chicken Pox	_____	_____	_____	_____	_____
Meningitis--------------------------	_____	_____	_____	_____	_____
Pneumonia	_____	_____	_____	_____	_____
Dizziness	_____	_____	_____	_____	_____
Recurrent Headaches	_____	_____	_____	_____	_____

Seizures --------------------------	____	____	____	____	_____
Encephalitis	____	____	____	____	_____
Epilepsy	____	____	____	____	_____
Diphtheria	____	____	____	____	_____
Whooping Cough	____	____	____	____	_____
Scarlet Fever ---------------------	____	____	____	____	_____
Anemia	____	____	____	____	_____
Head Trauma	____	____	____	____	_____

Other (please list) _____

Other (please list) _____

Does your child have allergies? ____Yes ____No

    If yes, what kind? _____

      Medication? _____ Age Diagnosed? _____

Has your child been hospitalized? ____Yes ____No

    If yes, note reason: _____ Age_____

Has your child taken any of the following?

	Yes	No	Duration of Medication	
Tofranil	____	____	____mo.	____yrs.
Dilantin	____	____	____mo.	____yrs.
Ritalin	____	____	____mo.	____yrs.
Mellaril	____	____	____mo.	____yrs.
Benadryl ---------------------------	____	____	____mo.	____yrs.
Thorazine	____	____	____mo.	____yrs.
Mysoline	____	____	____mo.	____yrs.
Dexadrine	____	____	____mo.	____yrs.
Other (please list)_____			____mo.	____yrs.
Other (please list)_____			____mo.	____yrs.

If drugs were used, have you seen a change in his/her behavior

____Yes ____No

Fig. 21 Central Auditory Disorder Case History (continued)

Has your child been placed on any special diets?

	Yes	No
Low Sodium	_____	_____
Low Sugar	_____	_____
Vegetarian	_____	_____
Food Color Diet	_____	_____
Weight Loss	_____	_____
Other (please list)_____	_____	_____

Since the diet, have you seen a change in his/her behavior? ____ Yes ____ No

---

Evaluation Record

Please note previous evaluations that your child has had:

	Yes	No	Age Evaluated	Results Normal	Irregular
Hearing Evaluations	____	____	_____	____	____
Neurologic (EEG, etc.)	____	____	_____	____	____
Psychological	____	____	_____	____	____
Intelligence Tests	____	____	_____	____	____
Speech and Language	____	____	_____	____	____
Vision	____	____	_____	____	____
Other (please list)_____				____	____

Social and Emotional Information

Please check whether or not your child has the following traits:

	Yes	No
Sensitive to loud sounds	____	____
Appears confused in noisy places	____	____
Follows and understands television programs	____	____
Easily Frustrated	____	____
Easily Distracted --	____	____
Hyperactive	____	____

Daydreams	_____	_____
Forgetful	_____	_____
Short attention span	_____	_____
Restless, problems sitting still ----------------------------------	_____	_____
Seeks attention	_____	_____
Disruptive	_____	_____
Rowdiness	_____	_____
Shy	_____	_____
Preference for playing with older children---------------------	_____	_____
Preference for playing with younger children	_____	_____
Headaches	_____	_____
Preference for solitary activities	_____	_____
Lacks self-confidence	_____	_____
Easily flustered or confused ------------------------------------	_____	_____
Temper tantrums	_____	_____
Problems following directions	_____	_____
Lacks motivation	_____	_____
Tires easily	_____	_____
Anxiety, tension ---	_____	_____
Disobedient	_____	_____
Uncooperative	_____	_____
Awkward, clumsy	_____	_____
Irritable	_____	_____
Impulsive --	_____	_____
Inappropriate social behavior	_____	_____
Destructive	_____	_____
Excessive talking	_____	_____
Easily upset by new situations	_____	_____
Does opposite of what is requested---------------------------	_____	_____

Fig. 21 Central Auditory Disorder Case History (continued)

Dislikes school	____	____
Does not complete assignments	____	____
Fakes illnesses	____	____
Has problems with time concept	____	____
Underachiever--	____	____
Problems with the law	____	____
Involved with alcohol	____	____
Involved with drugs	____	____
Had psychological counseling	____	____

Developmental History

What hand does your child prefer? ____ Right ____ Left ____ Ambidextrous

When did this preference occur? ____ Before 2 yrs. ____ After 2 yrs. ____ After 4 yrs.

At what age did your child learn to walk? ____ Before 1 yr. ____ After 1 ____ After 2

When did your child say his first word? ____ Before 1 yr. ____ After 1 ____ After 2

Educational History

Has your child ever repeated a grade? ____ Yes ____ No

If yes, why?_____

If yes, what grade?_____

Is your child:

	Yes	No
In an open classroom	____	____
In a traditional classroom	____	____
Receiving special help. If yes, type_____	____	____
Having problems with math	____	____
Having problems with spelling------------------------------------	____	____
Having problems with writing	____	____
Having problems with phonics	____	____
Having problems with science	____	____
Having problems with social studies	____	____

79

Having problems with foreign language   _____   _____

Having problems with reading --------------------------------- _____   _____

Other (please describe)_____   _____   _____

Does your child seem to rely more heavily on visual
    cues in school?   _____   _____

Have any relatives had difficulty learning in school?   _____   _____

      If yes, describe:_____

THANK YOU FOR YOUR HELP IN COMPLETING THIS QUESTIONNAIRE.

Fig. 21 Central Auditory Disorder Case History (continued)

requires precise and structured entries so that the information may be computer-programmed for the purpose of storage and subsequent analysis and retrieval. We take the opportunity at the time of the evaluation to engage the parent(s) in informal conversation. This forum is used to establish rapport with the family, give them a chance to express major concerns and feelings, and pursue history entries in greater detail.

The clinician needs to be very familiar with the case history form, so that the interview has continuity and focuses on the pertinent information related to the child's background. Typically, we do not include the child in the interview session. His presence during the discussion of his emotional difficulties, social problems, and academic struggles are not likely to promote a positive environment in which to conduct the subsequent evaluation. While there are certain instances in which it may be desirable to have the child present, clinicians must exercise good judgment when determining which parties should be involved in the history interview. Parents' concerns can also be of value in selecting appropriate tests for the CAP test battery. For example, it would help to avoid selecting tests that would penalize a child with limited vision, reading ability, or poor articulation. These concerns are directly addressed during the postevaluation counseling session, and suggestions are made to help the child, his parents, and teachers accommodate or adapt to the auditory problem. At that time, referral to professionals in other areas of expertise may be made.

COMPONENTS OF A CAPD CASE HISTORY

Myklebust (1954) has stressed the importance of having the first question of the case history relate to the parents' chief concern regarding their child. Addressing that information facilitates immediate rapport with the parents.

Certain types of information are common to most case histories for children. However, there are some questions that are unique to the child with a suspected CAPD. It is important to explore the child's hearing and speech history, maternal information, birth details, including prenatal, natal, and postnatal information, types of drugs mother and child have taken, various illnesses and accidents during childhood, special diets, social and environmental information, developmental factors, and educational history.

Prenatal, Natal, and Postnatal History. A history of prenatal problems and of natal and postnatal development often contributes helpful information about the causes of a central auditory problem. High-risk registers have been developed to aid the clinician in looking for possible peripheral hearing loss in children who manifest one or more of the high-risk factors. The High Risk Register, which is probably most commonly utilized by clinicians, is the one developed by the Joint Committee on Infant Hearing, comprised of representatives from the American Academy of Pediatrics, American Academy of Otolaryngology—Head and Neck Surgery, the American Nurses Association, and the American Speech-Language and Hearing Association (ASHA, 1982). Included on this register is a history of: (1) hereditary childhood hearing impairment; (2) congenital perinatal infection; (3) malformations of the head and neck; (4) birthweight less than 1500 grams; (5) hyperbilirubinemia exceeding level for exchange; (6) bacterial meningitis, and (7) severe asphyxia. These factors may be helpful in identifying children who may also be high risk for CAPD. For instance, a family history of deficient listening and/or linguistic skills together with maternal infection or stress, high bilirubin levels at the time of birth, and low birthweight may be indicators of central auditory problems. Precise, in-depth information concerning these factors has not been documented to date. However, it seems reasonable to assume that they may well be causes of CAPD.

Several examples of parallels between the causes of peripheral hearing loss and central auditory processing dysfunction can be made. For instance, Hall (1964) demonstrated that kittens that were asphyxiated showed more damage in the area of the cochlear nuclei of the brainstem than in the cochlea. Since anoxia and prematurity are often considered as having a direct relationship to one another (Gesell & Amatruda, 1947; Windle, 1950), a child born prematurely may also have damage to the cochlear nuclei. Therefore, these children may demonstrate difficulty in processing auditory information, especially in complex listening environments. Another possible indicator of a central auditory problem is Rh incompatibility, which results in kernicterus. Carhart (1967) noted that children who had hearing losses due to kernicterus may have decreased function in the central auditory pathways. Hardy (1961) had stated earlier that kernicterus is often associated with lesions at the level of the cochlear nuclei, low in the pons. He also suggested that lesions may occur at higher levels in the brainstem. Therefore, we should be alert to children who have suffered from Rh incompatibility and possible kernicterus, because such children may be at a high risk for central auditory dysfunction.

Heredity is another area of importance to explore in the case history. We have obtained CAPD histories in which more than one member of the child's family had difficulty processing auditory information. Subsequent evaluation confirmed that the child, one or more siblings, and one of the parents and/or grandparents had a central auditory problem. We also commonly hear remarks like, "His father has the same problem," and are convinced that hereditary factors are associated with central auditory dysfunction in some children. Table 8 shows the test results of members from three generations in one family who have CAPD, and all of whom failed the same tests.

Maternal conditions during pregnancy, such as diabetes, lues, radiation treatments, drug ingestions, and toxemia also should receive attention as possbile factors related to CANS involvement in the child.

Other factors to note regarding causation of CAPD may include the duration of pregnancy, duration of labor, and type of delivery. Gesell and Amatruda (1947) report that the duration of pregnancy seems to have some relationship to central nervous system damage. They note that the prevalence of such injury appears to be greater in children who are premature or postmature. These authors imply that prematurity may be related to intracranial hemorrhage. Postmature neonates may incur injury to their central nervous systems as the result of their increased size and, therefore, increased pressure on the brain during the birth process.

Table 8

Comparative CAP Scores in Percent on Family Members
Representing Three Generations

	Age	Competing Sentences L R	Filtered Speech L R	Binaural Fusion L R	Alternating Speech L R
Child	6.4	100– 0	70–52*	20*– 0*	90–100
Mother	31	100–100	66*–92	15*–70	100–100
Grandmother	60	100–100	64–38*	50*–58*	100–100

*Abnormal scores, either as a result of marked asymmetry between the ears or performance that fell below the range of scores for the age norm (CAP tests and their interpretation are discussed in Chapter 5).

Myklebust (1954) states that birth weights exceeding eight and one-half pounds or that are less than five and one-half pounds can be considered significant clinically. He also suggests that duration of labor may be associated with damage to the neonate at birth. Maternal labor, for a specific child, that is longer than average may be related to intracranial hemorrhage or anoxia. Similarly, he notes that labor that is very short in duration may also cause increased pressures that can result in intracranial hemorrhage.

Stander (1945) reports that the average length of labor depends on whether the child is firstborn or of subsequent birth order. He states that the average length of labor for firstborns is between fourteen and eighteen hours. Duration of labor for children born after the first child ranges from eight to twelve hours.

Breech births and caesarean deliveries are also important to consider when investigating the potential cause of a central auditory dysfunction. According to Myklebust (1954), breech birth can be associated with a difficult and long delivery in which injury may occur. The caesarean delivery may also be associated with accelerated adjustment to extrauterine life, which may cause an anoxic condition due to a change in the placental blood balance. The examiner should be aware that the cause of a caesarean delivery may be important. If long labor or respiratory difficulties of the neonate are the reasons for a caesarean, CANS difficulties may be more prevalent.

Other potential causes of LD and, perhaps, CAPD during pregnancy, or at the time of birth, may include: abnormal hormone secretions that affect brain cell development prior to birth (McEwen, 1983); maternal malnutrition during pregnancy, innate errors of metabolism (Simopoulos, 1983); maternal infections such as rubella, syphilis, cytomegaloviruses (CMV), herpes simplex, varicella (chicken pox), herpes zoster (shingles), toxoplasmosis, and tuberculosis (Sever, 1983); prenatal drugs (Gray & Yaffe, 1983); maternal smoking and alcohol intake (Streissguth, 1983), and obstetric medications used during the birth process (Broman, 1983).

CAPD may be the result of postnatal causes. Barr (1972) gives special mention to lead poisoning resulting from the ingestion of leadbased paints, eating and drinking from plates and cups with a high lead content, and breathing lead-laden air from automobile emissions. He states that this is particularly true among ghetto children, but offers no documentation. Needleman (1983) relates LD to toxicity from environmental pollutants such as lead, cadmium, methylmercury, and estrogen-like substances. Rimland and Larson (1983) analyzed 51 studies on hair mineral content and its relationship to "undesirable behaviors," which included LD, retardation, hyperactivity, delinquency, and others. They concluded that high levels of certain minerals, especially sodium, tend to be associated with undesirable behavior. There is some evidence to support the notion that noise levels in contemporary society may also contribute to the prevalence of CAPD. A review of this subject may be found in Mills (1975).

The role of childhood illnesses should also be examined in children with known or suspected central auditory dysfunction. Illnesses such as rubella, influenza, chickenpox, mumps, meningitis, encephalitis, anemia, and allergies should also be explored as possible causes of CAPD.

Hearing, Speech, and Language History.   The areas of hearing, speech, and language development and performance are crucial aspects of a central auditory case history. Information concerning ear infections, abscesses, and drainage is fundamental to proper evaluation of the problem. The belief that children with early, recurrent ear infections have a higher incidence of central auditory processing problems has received a great deal of attention in the professional literature. That literature, recently summarized by Webster (1983), presents conflicting views concerning this topic as it relates to CAPD. We will relate those views to our clinical experience in Chapter 8. We are confident that the occurrence of middle-ear infections during the critical period of language development has an adverse influence on the development of speech and language. Yet, how this relates to specific central auditory abilities in humans is a topic of some considerable controversy that needs further investigation.

We are in need of considerably greater data regarding speech and language development in children with confirmed central auditory disorders. For example, insight into the auditory learning skills of children with articulation disorders, children who are nonfluent, and those with aphasia and various language disorders is needed. Children with CAPD may have several subtle deviations in early speech and language development that may be overlooked until careful, ongoing analysis of their speech and language profiles is implemented.

Social and Emotional History.   Factors involving a child's social and emotional status are of great concern to parents and may be very helpful to the clinician in assessing his functional behavior. This information will often provide the diagnostician insight into whether the child has additional difficulties that may need to be investigated by other professionals such as counselors, psychologists, reading specialists, and speech-language pathologists. It will also aid the clinician in making appropriate suggestions for the functional management of the child's everyday environment. For example, if it is noted that the child has difficulty following directions, and the diagnostic results indicate that the youngster has a central auditory problem, special care should be taken to try to find ways to make it easier for the child to handle important directions at school and at home. Or, if the child is having difficulty managing necessary activities in his environment and has not developed successful coping behaviors, specific details of the problems should be elicited so that alternative behaviors can be recommended directly or with the cooperation of counselors or psychologists.

Developmental History. The developmental history generates information about the ages at which the child developed hand preference, learned to walk, and said his first words. This information is useful in determining whether the child matured according to normal developmental milestones.

Concerning laterality, Myklebust (1954) reports that children usually demonstrate a hand preference between the ages of 6 and 12 months and that it is usually fairly well established by the age of 18 months. He further states that disturbances in laterality are significant indicators of motor disorders. Gaddes (1978) has noted that learning problems are more common among left-handers with left hemisphere dysfunctions. Geschwind and Behand (1982) assert that hormonal imbalances may result in delayed growth or abnormalities of the left hemisphere, especially in males, and therefore contribute to greater frequency of left-handedness. This hormonal imbalance may thus account for the greater incidence of learning disabilities in males. At this point in time, we do not know if children with CAPD have a higher incidence of reversed, confused, or mixed laterality.* Such data have not been generated, since studies typically include only right-handed subjects and/or has not been established on children with documented CAPD. We are presently attempting to develop meaningful data on this subject.

The development of gross motor functions, such as sitting and walking, can also provide important information about a child's overall neurological integrity. The mean ages at which children sit alone and walk unsupported are 6 months and 13½ months, respectively (Myklebust, 1954). Documentation presently does not exist on how children with CAPD compare to these normal developmental milestones. As indicated in our history form, we are accumulating data on these factors as well.

The age at which a child says his first word may also give some indication as to whether he has difficulty perceiving spoken language. This is another area of behavior on which we currently have very poor data. The average age at which normal children say their first meaningful

---

*Mixed laterality is commonly defined as having a preference for the right hand and the left leg, or vice versa. Confused laterality is defined as a failure to demonstrate a preference for either hand.

word is approximately one year, but we do not presently know how the child with CAPD compares with that standard.

Educational History.   Concerns with academic performance and social relationships are expressed by parents, teachers, and psychologists as the primary reasons for referral for CAPD evaluations. Therefore, questions regarding the child's educational achievement are extremely important. Information regarding past and present performance often gives one increased insight into the ramifications of the child's disorder. It is important to know what grades the youngster is presently receiving, what subjects are most difficult and frustrating, when increased difficulty at school was first experienced, and the type of classroom structure in which the child is presently working. For instance, our experience has been that children with CAPD may do well in school up until about the third grade, at which level both instruction and language processes become more complex. Academic information may be presented more rapidly, and grading begins to receive greater emphasis. Such changes contribute to the child's frustration since he has progressively greater difficulty in handling his auditory world and begins to show unexpected difficulties in academic performance. It should be mentioned that we do see some children who are having auditory problems in kindergarten and first grade, evidenced primarily by poor communication efficiency and social demeanors. Information as to whether the child has been assigned to an open classroom environment, or has been placed in a structured, traditional room may alert the clinician to the demands placed on the child at school. Reports of subject matter with which the child has difficulty in school, together with the ways in which such material is presented, are often helpful in devising management and referral recommendations. We believe the educational history is a very important link to the ongoing study of CAPD in children. Many of these children are able to perform quite well in a variety of environments but still experience failure with academics.

5

Assessment Procedures

This chapter presents the major assessment techniques that are employed for defining central auditory function. The tests, used primarily by audiologists and speech-language pathologists, are quite different in nature and are utilized with different goals in mind. While emphasis is given to audiological tests employed in our hearing clinic over the past decade, nonaudiological measures that are in wide use are also reviewed. Thus, this chapter is designed to present our cumulative knowledge of the assessment in CAPD in children as well as to offer brief commentary on the state of the art in this country. The omission of some measures does not reflect on their quality but, rather, that they have not yet achieved sufficient recognition in the literature. Some of the tests discussed here are still experimental in nature. However, only in recent years have we begun to recognize CAPDs and have developed means to identify and define them. Thus, it seems likely that the future will bring new and better tests and/or refinements in the present measures. Nonetheless, the tests reviewed here have proved to be useful in the hands of competent and insightful clinicians.

NON-AUDIOLOGICAL ASSESSMENT

Numerous tests have been developed in attempts to measure the theoretical functions that comprise auditory perception. Their authors have widely divergent concepts of what is entailed in the process of audition and, consequently, today's commercially available tests have very different concepts and formats.

In order to appreciate the format of a test for assessing auditory processing, it is important to understand the author's concept of what process or processes are being measured. For example, Butler (1975) has separated the process of audition into the following elements: (1) recognition of intonation pattern; (2) short- and long-term memory; (3) closure;

(4) speech-sound discrimination; (5) auditory analysis, vigilance, and synthesis, and (6) association. Because of the numerous elements that Butler lists as parts of auditory processing, it is understandable that she feels a test that would provide a comprehensive evaluation of auditory perception would need to include some assessment of all of these areas. Many other investigators have developed terminology to explain their concepts of auditory perception processes. The majority of models for these processes are established on theoretical constructs of how audition relates to language functions. Some of the more popular tests of auditory perception will be presented together with the auditory processes they were designed to isolate and measure.

Illinois Test of Psycholinguistic Abilities.   Probably the best-known test that has been used to evaluate auditory perception is the Illinois Test of Psycholinguistic Abilities (ITPA), which was developed by Kirk et al (1968). This test contains 12 subtests that includes a battery of five auditory measures that are purported to assess functions of auditory sequential memory, association, reception, closure, and sound blending. This test was devised to focus on an examination of psycholinguistic abilities. The authors' concept of auditory perception was based on a theoretical model that included the above mentioned components of auditory skill, which they apparently felt could be isolated and measured. However, based on a factor analysis of the ITPA, Burns and Watson (1973) discovered that there was little or no support for the theory that the Revised Edition of the ITPA measures ten separate psycholinguistic abilities evaluated by 12 subtests. They further claimed that no more than five distinct abilities were measured with the ITPA and, if there were ten psycholinguistic entities, the test battery does not seem to be precise enough to isolate these functions. Burns and Watson also indicated that the five key areas that the ITPA does seem to measure assess auditory language ability instead of auditory processing ability. These results agree with those of Willeford (1976), who found that some children with confirmed central auditory disorders exhibit above average to average scores on all auditory subtests of the ITPA. Therefore, it appears that the ITPA may be measuring functions other than primary auditory functions. Moreover, McCarthy and McCarthy (1969) reported that performance patterns on subtests of the ITPA did not reliably differentiate children with learning disabilities from children who manifested other types of dysfunctions. Although the ITPA probably does serve some useful functions, the ability of this test battery to assess central auditory processing accurately should probably be reevaluated.

Lindamood Auditory Conceptualization Test.   The Lindamood Auditory Conceptualization (LAC) Test was designed to measure auditory

perceptual abilities (Lindamood & Lindamood, 1971). It can be administered to children of various chronological and mental ages functioning at
a range of academic attainment levels. The prerequisites of this test
consist of a child's ability to understand the concepts of same/different, to
discern the number concepts of one to four, and to be able to recognize
left-to-right direction. The test was designed to measure both speech-
sound discrimination and the ability to identify the number and order of
sounds spoken in various words. It was also conceived as a measure of
auditory perception that predicts the child's potential ability to read and
spell. Lindamood and Lindamood (1971) speculate that, since written
symbols portray various speech sounds, a child who has difficulty perceiving sound contrast and sound order in auditory stimuli will also have
difficulty reading and spelling.

Neither the ITPA nor the LAC test instructions specify that they
should be administered in a highly controlled test environment. Therefore, we presume that they can be given in any acoustic setting. In a pilot
study, Willeford and Mealler (1979) studied the effect of presenting the
LAC test on two non-CAPD children and three confirmed CAPD children
in controlled and noncontrolled backgrounds. They found that the CAPD
subjects obtained better scores when the test was given in a sound-proof
room but that the scores of the non-CAPD subjects did not differ in the
two test environments. It appears that the acoustic conditions of the
environment are very important when giving this and other tests that are
designed to measure auditory perception of speech. Therefore, tests that
are designed to measure auditory perceptual abilities but that do not
control the test environment may render spurious results that are dic-
tated by the acoustic factors present during the evaluation even though
test items may be repeated when environmental disturbances occur.

Goldman-Fristoe-Woodcock Auditory Skills Test Battery.   The Goldman-
Fristoe-Woodcock (GFW) Auditory Skills Test Battery (1974) is comprised
of a number of subtests that were developed to measure a variety of
auditory skills. As shown in Table 9, the test includes the following
subtest categories: (1) auditory selective attention test; (2) diagnostic
auditory discrimination tests, I, II, III; (3) auditory memory tests that
include recognition memory, memory for content, and memory for sequence, and (4) sound-symbol tests that include mimicry, recognition,
analysis, blending, speech symbol association, reading of symbols, and
spelling. The GFW tests are recorded on magnetic tape, which provides
playback consistency, and are available in either cassette or reel-to-reel
versions. Instructions direct the examiner to play the tapes at a "comfortably loud level," and to use them in a quiet environment on suitable tape
equipment. Unfortunately, it is left to each examiner's discretion to
decide what is "comfortably loud," "quiet," and "suitable." In spite of

Table 9
Goldman-Fristoe-Woodcock Auditory Skills Battery (1974)

1. Auditory Selective Attention Against Different Noise Backgrounds
2. Diagnostic Auditory Discrimination Tests I, II, III
3. Auditory Memory Tests
Recognition Memory
Memory for Content
Memory for Sequence
4. Sound Symbol Tests
Mimicry
Recognition
Analysis
Blending
Speech Symbol Association
Reading of Symbols
Spelling of Sounds

consistent taped stimuli, the lack of precision in any of the controls for auditory tests can lead to variability in test results.

Goldman, Fristoe, and Woodcock (1970) state that, ". . . . suspected deficits in speech-sound discrimination ability have been suggested by many writers to have profound effects upon an individual, particularly one who is developing oral and/or written language skills." That statement raises an interesting question about what constitutes a speech-sound discrimination deficit. We have evaluated many children with CAPDs who do not have speech discrimination problems per se or associated oral or written language difficulties, as we will describe in Chapter 7. However, we may well be dealing with a problem of semantics. That is, when a child has difficulty in understanding speech in a classroom or other social environment, it is more likely that he has a complex central auditory deficiency than a mere inability to make distinctions between phonemes. It is rare indeed to see children with CAPD who have speech discrimination problems as viewed from an audiological point of view.

The Auditory Selective Attention Test (1974) of the GFW was designed to be a simple but comprehensive measure of the ability to attend while listening in an increasingly intense noise background. This test consists of monosyllabic words presented with a signal-to-noise ratio ranging from +12 to −10 dB.

Schubert, Meyer, and Schmidt (1973) compared the performances for a group of normal young adults on the 1970 Goldman, Fristoe, Woodcock Auditory Discrimination Test (GFW), which was a forerunner of the 1974 auditory selective attention subtest, and Katz' Staggered Spondaic

Word (SSW) test. Their subjects scored in the normal range (91–99 percent) on the SSW, as expected, but from the first to the ninety-ninth percentile on the GFW. They concluded that there was essentially a "zero correlation" between test-retest performances on the noise subtest of the GFW and that they did not consider the test either reliable or valid as a measure of central auditory function.

The GFW Diagnostic Auditory Discrimination Test (1974) was devised in an attempt to assess an individual's ability to discriminate between speech sounds in quiet. The child in simply asked to select between two pictures in response to the spoken stimulus word.

The GFW Auditory Memory Test contains three separate subtests which purport to measure different aspects of short-term memory. Again, this test is presented on tape in quiet.

The Sound Symbol Test of the GFW includes assessment of such skills as mimicry, recognition, analysis, blending, speech symbols association, reading of symbols, and spelling of sounds.

The mimicry section is very interesting. The subject is requested to repeat test stimuli consisting of nonsense words. Hopefully, the examiner will be able to discriminate the client's responses. The test items include such nonsense words as "laift," "gubbest," and "fooch." The recognition subsection asks the subject to match spoken words with their picture representations. Initially, the stimuli consist of whole words such as "juice" but are subsequently presented one phoneme at a time, such as "j/...oo...s." The subject must point to the picture representing the word. Both mimicry and recognition subtests are difficult to distinguish from the auditory discrimination subtest.

The sound-analysis portion of the sound-symbols subtest consists of tasks in which the examinee is asked to identify from memory which sound in nonsense words is said first, second, and last.

Sound blending includes a task very similar to the sound recognition section. A word such as "t-ō-s-t" [toast] is sounded out and the child is asked to repeat the word he hears. It appears that the primary difference between a portion of the recognition test and the sound blending task is simply that in the recognition test the child is requested to point to a picture representing the word he hears.

The association section involves another interesting task. This test requires the child to associate a symbol with a nonsense word. Then, the new symbol with a new name is embedded in a group of symbols and the child must pick out the new symbol when its learned name is repeated.

The reading-of-symbols component of the sound-symbol subtest focuses on the subject's ability to sound out nonsense words such as "shum," "len," and "suss." The stimuli become progessively more difficult by including such nonsense words as "pelnidlun" and "bafmotbem."

Finally, the spelling-of-sounds section requires the child to spell nonsense words, such as "wifyep" and "depnonlel," presented via the test tape. The GFW sound-symbol test battery is summarized in Table 10.

The GFW's authors report that the reason for including the sound-symbol test is to "measure several basic abilities which are prerequisite to advanced language skills, including reading and spelling." They further state that, ". . . the GFW Sound-Symbol Test has been designed to identify subjects who are deficient in certain sound-symbol skills, and further, to describe this deficiency" (Goldman, Fristoe, & Woodcock, 1974).

It is interesting to note that the vast majority of subtests included in the GFW Test Battery include picture representations of the auditory target stimuli. Children who have a visual perceptual dysfunction, whether or not they have an auditory processing problem, may have difficulty identifying the stimulus through visual representation. Although this technique may be helpful for some children, the introduction of visual stimuli may confound the task of identifying an auditory problem.

The function of the central auditory nervous system is not addressed in this test battery. Rather, the test was designed to assess a series of theoretical auditory skills that may or may not be considered as clinical auditory perceptual functions, since no validation is provided.

Flowers-Costello Tests of Central Auditory Abilities. Flowers, Costello, and Small published the Flowers-Costello Test of Central Auditory Abili-

Table 10
Goldman-Fristoe-Woodcock Sound Symbol Tests (1974)

Test 1:	Sound Mimicry:	Measures the ability to imitate nonsense words.
Test 2:	Sound Recognition:	Measures the ability to recognize isolated sounds that comprise words.
Test 3:	Sound Analysis:	Measures the ability to identify various sounds of nonsense words.
Test 4:	Sound Blending:	Measures the ability to combine isolated sounds into meaningful words.
Test 5:	Sound Symbol Association:	Measures the ability to learn associations between nonsense words and visual symbols.
Test 6:	Reading of Symbols:	Measures the ability to make written-to-oral translations.
Test 7:	Spelling of Sounds:	Measures the ability to make oral-to-written translations.

ties (CAA) in 1970. This test battery is divided into two subtests purported to assess "selective or attentional" listening in young children. The subtests in the CAA test battery include a low-pass filtered speech (LPFS) test and a competing message (CM) test, both of which are recorded on a "single channel and presented to both ears." (Costello, 1977). According to Costello, the test was designed to permit early identification of children who have difficulty listening when the auditory stimulus is distorted or when competing messages are present. She states that the purpose of the test was "not . . . to locate or specify lesions in the auditory system." Rather, it was designed to identify children who have listening deficiencies that cannot be attributed to hearing loss, low intellect, or psychological problems (Costello, 1977). The test's authors claim that the LPFS test "represents the auditory perceptual factor of resistance to distortion," whereas it has been historically referred to as a site-of-lesion test for CNS involvement, specifically, for assessing contralateral temporal-lobe function (Bocca & Calearo, 1963; Lynn & Gilroy, 1975).

The first portion of the test consists of the LPFS subtest, in which 24 sentences are distorted by passing them through a low-pass filter cut off at 960 Hz. The child is requested to identify each test sentence by pointing to a picture representing the word that would complete the sentence.

The CM subtest of the CAA " represents the auditory perceptual factor of selective listening," which the authors define as, "the ability to select and differentiate a significant foreground stimulus from a nonrelevant background stimulus" (Flowers et al, 1970).

The CM test is also composed of 24 stimulus sentences that are recorded in such a way as to compete against a children's story. The two messages are mixed in one channel and presented to both ears simultaneously via earphones. This particular format represents diotic presentation of the stimuli as compared to the dichotic format of presenting the competing signals to different ears, which many researchers have used to assess temporal lobe function. The relative strengths of the two ears cannot be determined using the diotic format, although Jerger and Jerger (1975a) have shown via the SSI-ICM test, that this protocol is a measure of low brainstem integrity when the competing signals are directed to one ear at a time. Not only is the latter mode of presentation sensitive to CANS function, it can also be used to demonstrate ear differences, an important consideration in treatment strategy.

The authors of the CAA state that, "a child demonstrating difficulty in this central auditory ability will probably have difficulty in most areas of auditory perceptual function, and can be expected to manifest serious language development problems." (Flowers et al, 1970). Research supporting this statement has yet to be presented.

The test designers have selected a picture-pointing response for both subtests of the CAA. The child is instructed to point to one of three pictures representing a word that completed the stimulus sentence. As in the GFW, the implementation of the pictures during an auditory test may not be desirable, especially if the child has a visual perceptual dysfunction, or even poor visual acuity.

The CAA authors recommend that the subtests be administered in a quiet listening environment. They also suggest that loudness of the presentation level be calibrated prior to administering this test and they provide a means for doing so. These are positive recommendations and should be adhered to routinely by anyone who attempts to measure auditory skills.

Composite Auditory Perceptual Test. The Composite Auditory Perceptual Test (CAPT) (Butler, Hedrick, & Manning, 1973) is described by the authors as a test that can be utilized with grade-school children for assessing the "way in which . . . they perform on major perceptual processes." They further state that "perception is the immediate, short-term processing of information. It also involves attention, filtering out of irrelevant stimuli, memory, discrimination, and remembering things in order" (Butler et al, 1973).

One of the distinguishing features of the CAPT is that it can be administered by anyone who spends a little time with the manual; the authors state that no special training is needed. The CAPT is most appropriate for children in grades 1 through 3, but children in higher grade levels can also be tested with it. According to the authors, the CAPT assesses auditory abilities that they believe to be associated with early language development and important for classroom learning. They also report that the CAPT assesses "how well the listener can process information at the moment that he hears it" (Butler et al, 1973).

The CAPT consists of a three-part test that is recorded on tape. The recording can be transmitted via earphones or it is recommended that the children sit close to the tape recorder speaker. The authors do not suggest a loudness level for test presentation but do advise that the test be administered in a quiet environment.

The CAPT includes tests designed to meaure: (1) selective listening; (2) figure-ground discrimination for dissimilar voices; (3) figure-ground discrimination for similar voices; (4) temporal sequencing; (5) speech sound analysis; (6) consonant discrimination; (7) vowel discrimination; (8) auditory closure; (9) auditory synthesis; (10) syllable recognition; (11) discrimination of linguistic forms, and (12) discrimination of verb tense forms. As the reader can discern, the CAPT is a test designed to evaluate a series of auditory skills that are only thought to be important in auditory perception.

The CAPT manual indicate that, although the CAPT is a test of auditory perceptual abilities, the pictorial format of this test may be difficult for children with visual perceptual problems. However, suggestions are offered to circumvent that problem. As noted earlier, the utilization of visual stimuli as part of an auditory test can constitute a problem for test subjects.

Detroit Tests of Learning Aptitude.   The 19 subtests of the Detroit Tests of Learning Aptitude (DTLA) (Baker & Leland, 1967) are designed to evaluate overall functional learning ability. The authors recommend that individuals administering this battery have training in administering and interpreting psychological tests, so that the results obtained are "reliable and consistent" (Baker & Leland, 1967). However, Thurlow, and Ysseldyke (1979), as noted in Chapter 1, questioned the DTLA's reliability and validity.

The DTLA is normed on children and young adults from ages 3 to 19 years. The auditory subtests of the test battery are presented by live voice, with the intensity levels uncontrolled. The auditory and visual perceptual subtests are similar in format to the ITPA, both assessing theoretical concepts that the authors conceive to be important in auditory and visual perception.

The test manual for the DTLA includes a rationale for the significance of each subtest and offers guidelines for administering the tests.

In essence, the DTLA may have value for evaluating an individual's basic learning capabilities, but offer little help toward comprehensive evaluation of auditory perceptual skills.

Auditory Discrimination Test.   The Auditory Discrimination Test (ADT) was developed to measure "the ability to hear accurately" (Wepman, 1958). The child is presented with two words and is asked to indicate whether the words are the same or different. According to Wepman, every phonemic match that originates in the English language is paralleled within phonemic categories. In other words, phonemes within a select articulation category such as "simple stops" (*pool-tool*) are paired for the test stimuli.

Forty pairs of same or different words are presented by live voice. Only monosyllabic words are used, so that, according to the author, the test "avoids the possibility of discrimination being based on span rather than audition." Wepman suggests that this test is appropriate for children who are five to eight years of age, and reported that it has been found to be related to:

1. ability to develop speech accuracy
2. ability to read
3. ability to use phonics for reading
4. delay in developing speech based on auditory information
5. reading and speech difficulties
6. developing techniques for improving auditory perceptual skills
7. developing compensatory visual perceptual techniques while developing auditory skills

During the administration of the test, the child's back is turned to the examiner so that the child will not receive visual cues. The instructions suggest that the two words be read slowly and the child be given sufficient time to respond. Also, the examiner is instructed to read the words without emphasis or inflection, and at a level no louder than necessary. The instructions do not offer suggestions regarding specific loudness level of voice or mention environmental test conditions, such as the noise level of the test room.

Differentiation of Auditory Perceptual Skills. The Differentiation of Auditory Perceptual Skills (DAPS) Test (Reagan & Cunningham, 1976), another auditory perceptual skills test, is comprised of five subtests which include:

1. auditory cadence
2. auditory distinction
3. auditory imagery
4. syllable completion
5. auditory reasoning

The authors of this test feel that each area tested is important for perceiving auditory stimuli. This test of auditory perceptual skills is uncontrolled in terms of its acoustic format. Furthermore, the importance of these skills for auditory perception has not been validated. It seems to us that this test is a gross oversimplification of the complex processes involved in central auditory processing.

SUMMARY OF NONAUDIOLOGICAL EVALUATIONS

The foregoing tests typify non-audiological assessment instruments for children with suspected central auditory involvement. They are employed primarily by speech-language pathologists and other professionals, and are viewed from a perspective of assessing the auditory aspect of language performance. While it is unquestionably true that verbal signals trigger language processes, we still know little about the intricacies of that relationship. Moreover, that association becomes even more clouded when auditory tests, like most of those reviewed above, fail to control the variables of the test environment, acoustic characteristics of the test signals, consistency of the stimulus presentation speed and style, and often invoke the visual modality and cognitive demands. They largely ignore, or fail to detect and define, the individual's psychoneurological strengths. Rather, they attempt to measure psycholinguistic skills that incorporate numerous behaviors. Audiological tests of central function, conversely, minimize the dependence on linguistic talents and exercise the necessary test protocols that will permit assessment of the balance and strengths of the CANS.

AUDIOLOGICAL ASSESSMENT PROCEDURES

Audiological central auditory tests have been used primarily with adults for medical purposes to help confirm the presence and site of lesions in the CANS. Such tests are employed with children, however, to assess the "functional proficiency" of their CANS and with concern for its consequent effect on the development of academic, social, and communication skills. Even though many children demonstrate normal hearing for pure-tone and speech stimuli on standard audiological tests, they present unexplained difficulties with learning at school and/or with relating effectively to their families and friends, as noted earlier. Thus, the goal is to administer tests that will uniquely stress the auditory mechanisms at various levels of the central nervous system, with the objective of identifying deficiencies in an inefficient system. Such stress is created by special test design that requires more complex responses in the higher auditory centers than are necessary for responding to the awareness of a simple pure tone or for recognizing and/or repeating single spondaic or monosyllabic words. Even a defective CANS can process such stimuli with minimal difficulty. Thus, most central tests involve speech stimuli that have been modified in some fashion to make their understanding more difficult. Exceptions to the use of modified speech tests will be discussed in this chapter. The goal in all evaluations is to reveal a lack of ability that could account for the child's communication problems in difficult listening environments. While central auditory tests have different applications for adults and children, the principles and the nature of the tests are similar for both groups. However, certain test procedures are modified for children, and children's test norms are age-related. Tests discussed below are those that the authors and others have employed successfully with children. Some of these measures are experimental in nature, and one can recognize limitations in each of them. Collectively, they represent a series of techniques by which certain central auditory strengths and weaknesses can be identified and, as such, have been found useful for both experimental and clinical purposes.

Audiologists have successfully used with children a variety of central auditory tests that fall into four classifications: (1) tests in which speech stimuli are presented monotically (one ear at a time), including patterned or distorted verbal messages, messages that are embedded in competing signals, and pattern sequencing tasks with tones, the latter being a notable exception to the use of speech; (2) tests that present stimuli in a dichotic paradigm (different signals presented to the two ears at the same time; (3) tests that require the listener to sequence or sum complementary signals that are spatially separated in the two ears, and (4) electrophysiologic tests that objectively measure the physiologic response to auditory stimulation. The descriptions of these types of tests, listed in Table 11, illustrate the variety of strategies that seek to challenge the integrity of the CANS by subjecting it to stress in some unique fashion to provide a basis for comparing the performance of clinical populations with that of normal listeners. Modifications of verbal material are most widely used

Table 11
Central Auditory Processing Tests

Monotic Tests
    Frequency limited (filtered speech)
    Time altered (compressed speech)
    Pattern recognition (frequency)
    Performance-intensity function
    Ipsilateral competing signals (speech vs. speech or noise)
Dichotic Tests
    Competing digits
    Competing words (consonant-vowel-consonants, spondees)
    Nonsense sentences vs. discourse
    Real sentences vs. real sentences
    Competing consonant-vowels
Binaural Interaction Tests
    Binaural fusion
    Rapidly alternating speech
    Masking level differences
Electrophysiological Tests
    Aural reflex test
    Brainstem evoked response
    Cortical evoked response

---

for this purpose, because of the alterations that can be produced in the dynamic characteristics of speech signals as opposed to tones, white noise, and other signals. With speech signals, greater acoustical alterations can be exercised, while allowing the intelligibility of the signal to be maintained.

Audiological tests of CANS function are occasionally criticized as being insensitive for identifying auditory processing problems exhibited in "real life." According to Keith (1981), Butler believes that the strict controls and "artificial" test paradigms employed in audiological evaluations are less effective than are non-controlled tests that simulate natural listening situations. We believe, however, that the opposite is true. The very nature of many of the non-controlled tests, especially those that are "auditory-language" based, lend themselves to innumerable variables that undermine the ability to determine what auditory functions are being evaluated. As a result, our clinical experience with many children shows poor agreement between performance on non-controlled tests and rigidly controlled audiological tests. Although tested by a wide variety of noncontrolled assessment tools, many of our clientele are not diagnosed as having a CAPD until evaluated with rigorous, controlled, central auditory tests. Consequently, we maintain that a controlled auditory environment during an evaluation, using tests of CANS function, can more effectively uncover even the subtlest of CAPD.

A more direct response to Butler's criticism is that central auditory tests make no attempt to capture the listening realities of daily living. Rather, such tests seek only to assess the functional integrity of the auditory system. We hasten to add, moreover, that capturing the dynamic, infinitely changing auditory world on tape, or by any other means, is impossible. One can never lock the auditory world in time without altering its reality. Thus, the taping of auditory signals for a given test protocol merely seeks to lend consistency to the stimulus characteristics as opposed to live-voice tests in noncontrolled environments, which represent an unsatisfactory approach to measuring central auditory functions. We have found it interesting that many allied professionals will insist on the exacting controls of a sound-controlled test room, a calibrated audiometer, and a certified clinical audiologist when they are concerned about a child's peripheral auditory sensitivity. Paradoxically, such concerns are readily abandoned when they attempt to assess a child's central auditory status by live-voice protocols in uncontrolled acoustic environments. We submit that even greater care should be exercised for the evaluation conditions in central auditory disorders than for peripheral hearing impairment, since persons with central involvements are more vulnerable to the influences of ambient auditory signals. For one thing, peripheral hearing loss provides some insulation against the auditory background. For another, pure tones can be readily discerned in many competing environments in which grosser sounds do not mask a succinctly clear and simple pure tone stimulus, at least for tones above 250 Hz. Audiologists who have taken threshold measurements in industrial field settings to meet the guidelines of the Occupational Safety and Health Administration will confirm that faint pure tone signals are uniquely audible in the presence of seemingly greater noises of a grosser nature, particularly those above 500 Hz.

Because central auditory tests primarily contain speech signals that vary continuously and because one's ability to discriminate speech is diminished in competitive noise environments, CAP tests should be recorded on magnetic tape and played back under the rigorous conditions of precise loudness levels in acoustically-controlled test rooms. Thus, with the exception of electrophysiologic measures, the following tests describe several of the more widely used tests. All are recorded on magnetic tape. Factors that can alter the consistency of taped signals are addressed in the Appendix.

Monotic Tests

Monotic tests of central auditory function take a variety of forms, as shown in Table 12. The following discussion describes several of the more widely used tests.

Frequency limiting. Removing part of the frequency spectrum of speech stimuli limits their intelligibility, especially for persons with impaired temporal-lobe mechanisms. Limiting the frequencies of test stimuli may be achieved by passing the material through electronic filters that effectively eliminate high-frequency energy above a specific point. (Low-frequency elimination has not been found to be an effective clinical measure (Levy, 1981).) This technique has been validated on adults

Table 12
Monotic Tests*

Frequency Limiting—filtering out certain frequency content.
Time Altered—accelerating the rate of speech stimuli.
Performance-Intensity Functions—measuring intelligibility as a function of test
    intensity level.
Pattern Recognition—identification of changes in pitch.
Ipsilateral Competing Signals—intelligibility of speech in competition with
    speech or noise signals.

---

*Monotic tests present message(s) to only one ear.

suffering from temporal-lobe lesions. In such cases, poor performance is observed in the ear that is contralateral to the damaged hemisphere when compared with the performance of the ipsilateral ear, regardless of the side of cortical insult. It is this asymmetry between ears that generally confirms a cortical abnormality, since normal subjects show similar scores in both ears. However, reduced scores in each ear have been observed in certain patients. The reader is referred to Bocca, Calearo, and Cassinari (1954), Bocca and Calearo (1963), Lynn and Gilroy (1972), Lynn, Benitz, Eisenbrey, Gilroy, and Wilner (1972), and Lynn and Gilroy (1975, 1976, 1977) for discussions of the use of filtered speech and other measures of behavioral central tests on adults. The same pattern of results is often observed in children with central auditory problems (Willeford, 1976, 1977a, 1977b, 1980a; Willeford & Billger, 1978), although for obviously different reasons, since the great majority of such children do not have confirmed cortical insults. Table 13 presents the norms for the Willeford Filtered-Speech Test (1978b) on children ages five through ten years and for adults. The most notable feature in those data is an observable age progression, which suggests that task performance improves with maturation of the CANS. It may also be noted that performance is comparable in left and right ears and that a fairly wide range of scores is shown among subjects at all age levels. That is particularly true for younger children. As a result of that wide range, we consider scores of clinical patients as abnormal only when the scores for one or both ears fall below the range boundary for the patient's age or when there is an asymmetry (greater than 10–12 percent) between the scores for the two ears. We also

Table 13
Willeford Filtered Speech Norms (1978b)

Age	N	Mean LE − RE	Average Ear Difference*	SD LE − RE	Range LE − RE
5		Insufficient at present			
6	40	60.6–60.9	5.4	9.8–9.7	42/84–44/82
7	40	64.7–64.6	6.3	8.8–7.5	52/86–52/86
8	40	65.8–65.7	6.7	7.9–8.4	52/86–56/92
9	40	68.2–67.9	5.4	9.4–9.2	56/92–56/92
10	40	71.2–72.7	5.3	6.2–6.2	66/84–64/82
Adults[†]	20	87.6–87.4	0.2	6.3–5.7	74/98–74/98

*Only 18 of the 200 subjects had ear differences that exceeded 10 percent. The greatest difference in any subject was 16 percent that, in retrospect, probably reflected an abnormal auditory sustem.
[†]College students; ages 18–29 years (Ivey, 1969).

believe that the practice employed by some audiologists of labeling as abnormal those scores that fall below one standard deviation is questionable, since one-third of the subjects used in the norming exercise performed below that level. Table 14 presents the performances of a series of young subjects, each with histories of auditory, academic, social, and/or emotional difficulties. They all should be achieving scores better than the lowest score in their age range and have comparable results in each ear. We should remind the reader that these, and all other subjects discussed in this book, have normal hearing on non-CAP tests. All subjects in the Table, except number seven, show asymmetries between ears or have poor scores in both ears.

Table 15 presents the filtered speech scores of four younger children who illustrate the heterogeneity of results that can be seen among children with subtle CAP disorders. These youngsters were poor listeners both in and out of the classroom and were referred by school personnel for that reason. The test results of these patients are included to show that the filtered speech test is one that some children with central auditory dysfunctions can perform quite well. Individual performances on this and other tasks of central auditory function vary widely. This fact emphasizes that central auditory disorders may be manifest in the reduction of any one of many skills, since all levels of the central auditory nervous system and its corresponding mechanisms and/or functions should be susceptible to disorder, a condition that undoubtedly contributes to the heterogeneity of this population. In summary, it would be naive to believe that any single test would capably identify every child with a central auditory disorder.

Table 14
Clinical Results of Filtered Speech Tests on
Youngsters with Academic,
Auditory, and Social Difficulties

			Filtered Speech Score	
Subject	Age	Sex	LE	RE
1	9	M	58%	84%
2*	10	F	34%	60%
3	13	M	54%	74%
4	14	M	22%	38%
5	16	F	18%	20%
6	18	M	32%	32%
7†	9	M	92%	84%

*Only subject with a diagnosed language disorder. All subjects except No. 3 failed from 1 to 4 additional CAP tests as well.
†Passed three other CAP tests as well, but failed a fourth.

Table 15
Filtered Speech Results on a Group of Children with
Academic, Auditory, and Social Difficulties

			Filtered Speech Score	
Subject	Age	Sex	LE	RE
SP*	6.6	M	0%	0%
DM*	6.7	M	0%	0%
OW*	10	M	12%	16%
DM†	6.5	M	70%	72%

*Also failed three other CAP tests.
†Only CAP test passed out of four tests administered.

Compressed speech. Compressed, or accelerated, speech is also a central auditory test applicable for children. It capitalizes on the fact that a disturbed temporal (time) factor is a characteristic that has been demonstrated in certain persons with cortical auditory disorders. Compressed speech involves the use of "speeded-up" recorded speech material in which the frequency spectrum of the presentation is held constant. The most commonly used compression rate has been 60 percent. Thus, the peculiar vocal distortions (the "chipmunk" quality) that accompany standard speech recordings when they are played back at rates faster than those at which they were recorded are avoided. Beasley and Freeman (1977) present a review of the rationale for the development and use of compressed speech for diagnostic purposes. The technique has been utilized in numerous studies to establish its relationship to such factors as hearing impairment (Kurdziel, Rintelmann, & Beasley. 1975), articulation disorders (Orchik & Oelschlaeger, 1974), reading deficiencies (Freeman & Beasley, 1976), auditory processing problems (Heard et al, reported by Beasley & Freeman, 1977), aging (Konkle & Bess, 1974), and cortical lesions (Kurdziel Noffsinger, & Olsen, 1976). We have used compressed speech tests developed by Beasley, Maki, and Orchick (1976)* with many children as a supplement to the Willeford Test Battery (Willeford, 1976; 1980a)† and other tests we use to evaluate children with suspected central auditory dysfunction at Colorado State University. Compressed speech is a measure that assesses a facet of CANS function that other tests do not.

---

*Versions from a variety of recorded speech materials and several compression rates are not commercially promoted, but are available on request from Daniel Beasley, Ph.D., 807 Jefferson Ave., Memphis, TN.
†Available from Jack Willeford, Ph.D., 1013 Valleyview Road, Fort Collins, CO 80524. This battery is also available on request only, and not available through commercial outlets.

Table 16

Comparisons of Central Auditory Test Results among
Children with Central Auditory Dysfunctions. Tests Include
Willeford Battery* and Compressed WIPI (CW)
(Compression Rate was 60%; SL = 32 dB SL).

Subject	Test				
(Sex-Age)	CS	FS	BF	AS	CW
CT	L-80	58**	35[+]	100	68[‡]
(M—9.0)	R-100	84	45[+]	100	76[‡]
MP	L-80	52**	30[+]	100	52[‡]
(F—8)	R-80[+]	64	40[+]	100	60[‡]
HS	L-90	68	85	100	54[‡]
(M—9)	R-100	66	85	100	58[‡]
BH	L-90	62**	45[+]	80[+]	96
(F—10)	R-50[+]	48**	50[+]	70[+]	96

*Competing (dichotic) sentences (CS), filtered speech (FS), binaural fusion (BF), and alternating speech (AS).
[+]Abnormal response (below normal range for age level).
[‡]Poor performance in relation to mean scores reported by Maki, Beasley, and Orchik, 1973.

Table 16 presents the clinical results on a group of children using the compressed WIPI tests and the Willeford Battery. Observe that there is no apparent pattern to the tests on which failures occur. Compressed speech was the only test one child could not perform adequately, whereas another failed all of the tests except compressed speech. Such results in our clinical experience, we believe, confirm the suspicion that children with central auditory dysfunctions form a diverse group of individuals who can only be evaluated properly by a comprehensive series of tasks. It is also this very fact that argues against using group data to study central auditory phenomena since given individuals can skew data sharply when their scores are averaged.

Pitch Pattern Sequence Test.   The Pitch Pattern Sequence Test (PPST) was developed by Pinheiro (1977a)[‡] for the assessment of CAPD. It has both child and adult versions. The uniqueness of this test lies in the facts that it employs nonverbal stimuli and assesses both pattern-perception skill and temporal-sequencing ability. The children's version requires the subject to report the "high-low" patterns of the presentation of three 500 msec tones separated by 300 msec intervals. The tone frequencies are 880 Hz (low) and 1430 Hz (high), which are played in six different combinations: HLH, LHL, HHL, LLH, HLL, and LHH. The test has provisions for training the subject with 20 practice pairs (LH and HL) and each ear may

[‡]Test available from Auditec of St. Louis, 330 Selma Avenue, St. Louis, MO 63119.

be tested under earphones with 25 to 60 three-tone patterns presented to each ear separately. The test may also be presented in soundfield, but a great deal of information is lost when subjects are tested binaurally. The test also features multiple response modes; that is, subjects may respond by whistling or humming the pattern perceived, reporting it verbally, or pointing to or tapping high and low objects such as books or boxes. Performance differences are not observed between response methods in normal subjects. However, it has been shown that subjects with cortical lesions (Musiek & Geurkink, 1980; Musiek, Geurkink, & Keitel, 1982; Pinheiro, 1978) are only able to perform the hummed response and score poorly when required to respond verbally or manually. A similar result has been observed in split-brain patients who could perform all response modes prior to surgery (Musiek, Pinheiro, & Wilson, 1980; Musiek, Wilson, & Reeves, 1981). Table 17 presents the PPST results of 14 young children with learning disabilities (Pinheiro, 1977b). Once again, considerable heterogeneity may be seen in these subjects, but their results suggest that the PPST is a very sensitive measure when its group data is compared with a series of other tests. These data should also be considered in the light of differences in the age norms for each test rather than the fixed values shown in this table.

Performance-Intensity Functions. Jerger (1981) demonstrated the appropriateness of performance-intensity functions for phonetically-

Table 17

Mean Central Auditory Test Results on 14 Children with Learning Disabilities; Tests Include Pitch Patterns, the SSW, and the Willeford Battery

	Left Ear	Right Ear	Norms*
Alternating Speech	94	96	80/100
Binaural Fusion	62	72	75/100
Low-Pass Filtered Speech	68	75	70/100
SSW (Alternating)	89	97	80/100
SSW (Simultaneous)	75	88	75/100
Competing Sentences	71	95	80/100
Simultaneous Sentences	38	71	75/100
Pitch Pattern Sequence Test (Verbal)	22	23	75/100
Pitch Pattern Sequence Test (Hummed)	93	88	90/100

Adapted from Pinheiro, M. Auditory pattern perception in patients with left and right hemisphere lesions. *Ohio Journal of Speech and Hearing,* 1977a, *12,* 9–20. With permission.
*Norms are not based on age-specific values.

balanced words (PI-PB) with children having either brainstem or temporal lobe dysfunction. She noted that brainstem disorders showed more
dramatic results. This test can probably be given to any child who can
perform a speech discrimination test, but it is time consuming. It involves
presenting the test stimuli at increasing sensation levels in search of the
rollover phenomenon (Jerger & Jerger, 1971).

Synthetic Sentence Identification-Ipsilateral Competing Message Test.
The Synthetic Sentence Identification-Ipsilateral Competing Message
Test (SSI-ICM) (Jerger & Jerger, 1974, 1975a) is a test of brainstem integrity that is comprised of nonsense sentence stimuli that are third-order
approximations of real language competing with a historical recitation
about the life of Davy Crockett. These are presented at progressively
difficult sentence-to-competition ratios. We have used this test with
several children but have found that it is limited by the requirement that
the subjects be able to read (or recognize) the correct item from randomly-
ordered lists of ten nonsense sentences. Since some children are learning
disabled for vision or reading, or have not developed adequate reading
skills, the SSI-ICM is not an appropriate test for this population. One
could simply have the child repeat what he hears but since the stimulus
language is meaningless, it would be a difficult task for the child and a
problem to score. Jerger has, however, reported successful use of the
SSI-ICM with children (1981).

Speech-in-Noise. Speech discrimination measured against a competition of noise is a monotic test technique that may be used with
children, but it has received relatively little attention in the literature. This
technique is useful when administered in a monotic mode employing
white noise at a signal-to-noise ratio of 0 dB. The works of Olsen, Noffsinger, and Kurdziel (1975), Sinha (1959), Noffsinger, Olsen, Carhart, Hart
and Sahgal (1972), and Morales-Garcia and Poole (1972) should serve as
the procedural protocols. These studies have all suggested that speech
discrimination in the presence of monotically presented noise, decreases
with both brainstem and temporal-lobe involvements. This procedure is
valuable in that it may indicate an asymmetry between ears and, therefore, CANS asymmetry. Such knowledge has important implications for
management as discussed in Chapter 6. However, speech-in-noise testing is often administered binaurally under earphones or in soundfield.
When such modifications in procedure are made, the sensitivity of this
test diminishes substantially because it nullifies the ability to isolate each
ear's CANS function. Detailed reviews of speech-in-noise measures as
tests for central auditory dysfunction have been presented by Willeford
and Billger (1978) and McCroskey and Kasten (1980). Regardless of which

monotic test(s) a clinician may choose to employ, they have the advantage of requiring relatively simple instrumentation such as that found in dual-channel audiometers and tape recorders.

Dichotic Tests.

Dichotic tests, listed in Table 18, utilize a variety of techniques and stimulus materials, which are also quite effective for evaluating central auditory functions in children. These tests are thought to primarily stress the temporal lobes. Dichotic protocol pits a signal presented to one ear against a different signal simultaneously presented to the opposite ear, and the listener is asked to repeat the signal in one or both ears. The two-ear procedure usually involves signals presented at equivalent loudness levels, whereas the single-ear procedure may be arranged in various signal-to-competition ratios. Dichotic tests require one and a half or two-channel audiometers and stereo tape decks. The following tests are those that either the present authors or others have found applicable and useful with children.

Digits. In this technique, different pairs of numbers are presented simultaneously to the two ears. For example, the numbers five and nine may be presented to the subject's right ear at the same time the numbers two and eight are presented to the left ear. The subject is asked to repeat all of the numbers heard, if possible, using any strategy of his choice. A perfect response would be to repeat all four numbers. Although digits have been employed experimentally and clinically for many years, their effective clinical utilization with children has only recently been reported by Musiek et al (1982).

Table 19 shows the results of three dichotic tests, including digits, on a series of children reported by Musiek and Guerkink (1980). It is appar-

Table 18
Dichotic Tests*

Digits—different digits, presented in competition.
Words (CVCs—spondees)—monosyllabic or bisyllabic words presented in competition.
Nonsense Sentences vs. Discourse—nonsense sentences competing against continuous discourse.
Real Sentences vs. Real Sentences.
Consonant Vowels (CVs)—different CV pairs in competition.

*Dichotic tests present different messages to the two ears simultaneously. In some test designs the listener is required to repeat both messages. In others, response is to one ear only while attempting to ignore the competing message in the other ear. Test protocols vary widely in terms of message-to-competition ratios.

Table 19

Results of Dichotic Digit Test, Willeford's Dichotic Sentences,
and the SSW

Sub-ject	Age	Sex	Dichotic Test Scores*					
			Digits		Sentences		SSW	
			L	R	L	R	L	R
1	9	M	35[†]	80[†]	40[†]	80[†]	50[†]	78[†]
2	8	M	65[†]	85	0[†]	100	5[†]	85[†]
3	9	F	92	96	50[†]	95	78[†]	96
4	9	M	90	88	55[†]	100	82[†]	82[†]

Adapted from Musiek, F & Geurkink, N. Auditory perceptual problems in children: considerations for the otolaryngologist and audiologist. *Laryngoscope*, 1980, *90*, 962–971. With permission.
*Approximated from graphs.
[†]Abnormal responses.

ent that any of the three tests would have identified a central auditory problem in the first two youngsters. However, it may be seen in the results of the other two children that such tests are not equally sensitive for all children with central auditory disorders. Diversity of results may be anticipated, since these tests are sufficiently different in a number of aspects to represent rather different linguistic/auditory tasks, even though they all employ some form of dichotic paradigm. A comtempo-rary review of dichotic digit tests attests to their wide usage, albeit chiefly with adults (Musiek, 1983).

Staggered Spondaic Word Test. A great deal has been written about the Staggered Spondaic Word (SSW) Test (Katz, 1962; 1968) for use with both adults and children. It is designed so that two spondaic words[§] partially overlap. The second syllable of the first spondee word, which originates in one ear, occurs nearly simultaneously with the first syllable of the second spondee word, which originates in the opposite ear. The subject is simply asked to repeat the spondee words presented to the two ears. The following is an example of the test protocol.

	Non-Competing	Competing	Non-Competing
RE	out	side	
LE		in	law

[§]Spondaic words are two-syllable words presented so that each syllable has equal stress. For example, "cow-boy."

Much of the information about this test (available from Auditec of St. Louis, cited earlier) concerns its use as a diagnostic measure for assessing central lesions in adults (Brunt, 1978). More recently, however, it is being used in a modified form with children. Presentations of selected studies related to use of the SSW have been compiled in a recent book (Arnst & Katz, 1982), which contains a number of reports that appear to support the value of the SSW as a measure for assessing central disorders in children. The reader is also referred to other studies of the SSW (Dempsey, 1977; Johnson, Enfield, & Sherman, 1981; Musiek et al, 1982; Musiek & Guerkink, 1980; Pinheiro, 1977b; Sweitzer, 1977; White, 1977; et al, 1982).

Synthetic Sentence Identification-Contralateral Competing Message. The clinical use of the SSI test in the ipsilateral mode (SSI-ICM) was presented earlier under the discussion of monotic tests. However, it can be presented in a dichotic or contralateral mode (SSI-CCM). This test may also be given to children (Jerger, 1981). However, there are other measures that are easier, more practical, and less time consuming. The Jergers concede that the SSW is more sensitive than the SSI-CCM, and therefore may be preferable for identifying temporal-lobe disorders in adult patients (Jerger & Jerger, 1975a).

Real Sentences. A dichotic test using actual sentences was developed by Willeford in 1968 and validated initially on adults with cortical lesions (Lynn & Gilroy, 1975, 1976, 1977). This test is now being used with children in a variety of professional settings (Musiek & Guerkink, 1980; Musiek et al, 1982; Pinheiro, 1977b; Willeford, 1976; 1977a; 1977b; 1978a; 1978b; 1980a; Willeford & Billger, 1978). It is one of the tests in a four-test battery of central auditory tests. The filtered speech test described earlier constitutes a second test in the battery. The other two tests, binaural fusion and alternating speech, will be discussed subsequently. The test protocol with dichotic competing sentences is to present different sentences that are of similar length and semantic content to each of the subject's ears; for example, "I read that in the newspaper" versus "The man on the radio said it." The test may be administered by presenting one sentence from pairs of sentences to the test ear at 35 dB SL while the non-test ear receives the other sentence from the pair at 50 dB SL. The latter serves as the competition, and the subject is asked to not listen to it.

An occasional comment about the Willeford Competing Sentence Test is that it places inordinate dependence on memory and, thus, clouds interpretation of results. While that would more likely be true for sentences than for briefer stimulus material, abnormal performance on this test is most commonly manifested as a failure to perform in one ear only.

We are not aware of any evidence that auditory memory is stronger for signals heard in one ear as opposed to the other. Furthermore, our experience has been that when a person has difficulty understanding these sentences in only one ear, this individual responds normally in that same ear when the competition is removed. However, if a child has trouble repeating sentence-type material in the absence of competition, a significant language dysfunction may be strongly suspected. Tests of shorter item length would appear to be more appropriate as diagnostic instruments in such cases. It seems reasonable to conclude that if a child can correctly repeat sentences without competition that decreased performance on dichotic sentence tests is the result of faulty auditory input rather than one of memory dysfunction.

An alternative test option is to present both sentences in each pair at 50 dB SL, again one sentence to each ear, and instruct the subject to attempt to repeat both of them. This task proves to be more difficult for many subjects, and memory may influence test performance. Single and double-ear response norms are presented in Tables 20 and 21, respectively. As with many central auditory tests, both response norms show improved performance as a function of age.

Ipsilateral-Contralateral Competing Sentence Test. The authors have recently developed another natural-sentence test, which was designed to circumvent certain limitations of other tests and to provide a comprehensive task paradigm. The resulting product was the Ipsilateral-Contralateral Competing Sentence (IC-CS) Test. The IC-CS is based on certain features of the SSI concept, except that it avoids requiring the subject to read, uses real sentences as both stimulus and competition items, and it is not a closed-set procedure. The test consists of five sets of ten-sentence pairs, one sentence in each pair spoken by a female voice, the other by a male voice, in the following test protocols:

Contralateral Competing Sentences (CCS)

List A—Male and female voices presented to opposite ears. Response is required to the female voice in the test ear, presented at 35 dB SL (Re: pure tone average (PTA)), while the male-voice competition is supplied to the non-test ear at 50 dB SL. Signal-to-competition ratio (SCR) is -15 dB.

List B—The test and competition ears are reversed and the other ear is tested for reception of the female voice. The same SCR is used.

List C—Male and female voices are presented to opposite ears at 50 dB SL in each ear (SCR = 0 dB). Subject is instructed to repeat both sentences.

Ipsilateral Competing Sentences (ICS)

Table 20
Norms for Willeford Competing Sentences
(Unilateral Response)

Age	N	Expected Result		Mean		SD		Range	
		Weak Ear	Strong* Ear	Weak Ear	Strong* Ear	Weak Ear	Strong* Ear	Weak Ear	Strong* Ear
5	25	20–90/100		24.8–	9.4	35.9–4.4		0/80–90/100	
6	40	60–90/100		59.5–96.5		33.2–4.0		0/100–90/100	
7	40	70–100		67.8–97.5		31.2–3.6		0/100–90/100	
8	40	80–100		83.0–98.0		22.2–3.2		10/100–90/100	
9	40	90–100		93.0–98.8		9.8–2.6		70/100–90/100	
10	40	100–100		98.4–99.2		3.6–2.6		90/100–90/100	
5/10	40	70–100		71.6–95.9		22.7–3.5		0/100–90/100	

*Strong ears were predominantly right ears. Left ears were the strong ears in only 13 of the 225 subjects.

Table 21
Norms for Willeford Competing Sentences, Bilateral-Response
(N = 20 at each age level)

Age	Score*	Range	Mean Ear Response Order[†] L	R
6-year-olds	46.0%	20/70%	3.5	6.5
7-year-olds[‡]	54.5%	30/80%	3.5	6.5
8-year-olds	62.8%	45/100%	3.6	6.4
9-year-olds	73.0%	45/90%	3.7	6.3
10-year-olds	80.5%	50/100%	4.3	5.7
11-year-olds	83.5%	65/100%	5.1	4.9
12-year-olds	85.3%	65/100%	4.8	5.2

*Single-correct responses = 5%. Double-correct responses = 10%.
[†]Ear stimulus to which subject responded first.
[‡]7-year-old data is interpolated.

List D—Both sentences are presented to the same ear (left or right). Response is to the female voice as in Lists A and B. The SCR = 0 for this procedure (female voice at 50 dB SL and the male voice at 50 dB SL) when given to children under the age of twelve. In older children and adults, the SCR = −5 (female voice at 45 dB SL and the male voice at 50 dB SL).

List E—The same procedure as in List D is now conducted in the subject's other ear.

As in the Willeford Competing Sentence Test, the sentences have similar length, but each competing pair includes one common word that is offset from its counterpart by one syllable. That is, they do not begin and end at the same time. The purpose was to make them semantically more competitive by allowing both ears to hear the common word. The present IC-CS norms are shown in Table 22. Plans include expanding these norms, developing norms for the male voice, and for a number of other variations in the test procedure, such as norming each test list for each of the five test protocols.

As shown in the earlier discussion of dichotic sentences, the contra-lateral (dichotic) test conditions would primarily challenge the integrity of the auditory regions of the cortex, according to studies on adults, whereas the ipsilateral conditions specified for Lists D and E most likely challenge the proficiency of the brainstem as found with the SSI-ICM (Jerger & Jerger, 1975b).

Scoring for the IC-CS is based upon the degree to which the language in, and meaning of, each test item is preserved; that is, without being adversely influenced by the competition sentence in any substantial way. For example, two errors per sentence of any of the following combinations constitutes an incorrect response:

Table 22

Norms in Percent for the Willeford-Burleigh Ipsilateral-Contralateral Competing Sentence Test

Age		Test List				
		A	B	C	D	E
6 & 7 (N = 27)	Mean	81.5	89.6	44.8	82.6	87.0
	S.D.	13.2	9.8	11.3	12.6	9.9
	Range	50/100	70/100	30/75	60/100	70/100
8 & 9 (N = 27)	Mean	89.6	90.4	61.9	85.5	92.6
	S.D.	10.6	12.9	12.7	10.9	9.8
	Range	60/100	60/100	40/85	60/100	70/100
10 & 11 (N = 27)	Mean	93.0	94.1	70.0	96.7	97.0
	S.D.	7.8	8.9	11.2	4.8	5.4
	Range	80/100	70/100	50/85	90/100	80/100
12-adult (N = 27)	Mean	98.2	99.3	83.7	96.9	96.3
	S.D.	4.0	2.7	9.1	6.9	6.3
	Range	90/100	90/100	65/100	80/100	80/100

1. Borrowing from a competing sentence
2. Omitting a word
3. Adding a word
4. Substituting a word not found in either sentence, or
5. Any single word error that alters the meaning or intent of the sentence

The IC-CS norms were intriguing in the sense that no left-right ear differences were observed for presentations in the contralateral mode, as found with younger children on the Willeford Competing Sentence Test and on other central auditory tests. However, scores did improve with age, and the range of scores diminished. The reason why ear differences were not observed on CCS Lists A and B is not clear. That is, they may not offer the same degree of competition presented by the same voice uttering different sentences. Obviously, different acoustic features would be involved in the task to some degree.

Table 23 presents clinical results with the IC-CS on a series of patients. The nine-year-old subject (DS) is a very interesting case. He scores poorly on the IC-CS and six other CAP tests, yet he has developed sufficient compensatory skills to survive quite well at school, except in classes where group discussion is required and in complex social environments. We are continuing to evaluate the IC-CS, since it offers a variety of challenges for the CANS and is easily and quickly administered.

Consonant-Vowel Test. Dichotic Consonant-Vowel (CV) tests have been widely used for experimental purposes, and summaries of this work may be found in the proceedings of a Symposium on Central Auditory Processing Disorders at the University of Nebraska Medical Center (1975) and in Berlin and McNeil (1976). The test protocol involves presenting a CV, such as /ba/ to one ear while a different CV, such as /da/, is presented to the other ear. There are six CV stimulus items (pa-ba-ta-da-ga-ka) that occur in all possible combinations and arranged in 30 paired items per test list. The subject is requested to repeat what is heard in both ears. The test is scored for correct items in the left ear, right ear, and both ears. A CV test has also been normed for children 5–13 years of age (Berlin, Hughes, Lowe-Bell and Berlin, 1973). However, on the basis of surveys by Katz (1978a) and by Willeford (1980b), CV tests are apparently not used on a regular basis for clinical purposes. Although they, and others, have found this test to be very sensitive, Lynn and Gilroy (1977) note that "for most patients with brain tumors we have found that the dichotic CV test is often very difficult, and we usually use it only in selected cases with excellent hearing levels and minimal neurological deficit."

Table 23
Ipsilateral-Contralateral Competing Sentence Test Results
in Percent for Patients with CAPD

Subject/ Age	Ear	Contra- lateral Score	Ipsi- lateral Score
	L	20*	20*
EW/7	R	50*	0*
	Bilateral	20*	
	L	20*	60*
DS/9	R	100	30*
	Bilateral	45*	
	L	10*	80
JH/11	R	90	80
	Bilateral	45*	
	L	—	30*
TH/24	R	—	30*
	Bilateral	—	
	L	—	30*/20*†
RF/27	R	—	30*/30*†
	Bilateral	—	
	L	60*	30*
CB/35	R	70*	60*
	Bilateral	70	

*Abnormal response.
—Did not test.
†Test repeated six months later.

Binaural Interaction Tests.

Binaural interaction tests of central auditory function, which are described below, take a variety of forms, as shown in Table 24.

Binaural Fusion. Binaural fusion may qualify as a dichotic listening test in the sense that the two ears are simultaneously stimulated with different signals. However, in binaural fusion the signals involve complementary acoustic components of the *same* stimulus words as opposed to competing components. Specifically, one ear receives selected high-frequency energy of a given word while the other ear receives selected low-frequency energy of that same word. Thus, we consider it more appropriate to include it under binaural interaction tasks. The principle of the test is for the high and low frequency components of the words, both

Table 24
Binaural Interaction Tests

Binaural Fusion—combining high-frequency bands in one ear with low-frequency bands of the same signal in the other ear.
Rapidly Alternating Speech—bursts of continuous sequential signals alternating between the two ears.
Masking Level Differences—comparison of two binaural signals when in and out of phase.

difficult to discriminate when presented individually, to be synthesized into a relatively intelligible message when presented simultaneously as their collective acoustic components are fused into meaningful words by the brainstem system. Matzker (1959) first described the concept of this test, and it has since been molded into a variety of test protocols by Linden (1964), Smith and Resnick (1972), Ivey (1969), Willeford (1976, 1980a), Willeford and Billger (1978), Pinheiro (1977b), and Musiek et al (1982). Alterations in the test include type of stimulus words employed (bisyllabic words and monosyllabic words), width of pass-bands, frequency region of pass-bands, and sensation levels at which the bands are played. While this type of test seems capable of identifying brainstem dysfunction, its sensitive stimuli are influenced by all of the foregoing factors, as well as by peripheral hearing loss, accuracy of pure tone threshold measurements on which the test SLs are set, and by the care and use of the tapes themselves and their playback units. Of course, those factors are important considerations in administering any taped test, but they are especially critical for tests of CVs, binaural fusion, filtered speech, compressed speech, or any other technique that represents a reduction in the normal redundancy of spoken language. This test is the third measure in the Willeford Test Battery. Its stimuli were generated by Ivey in 1969. Its norms are shown in Table 25; as in previous test norms, some degree of improvement with age may be observed.

Rapidly Alternating Speech. This is a test in which verbal stimuli are alternately switched from ear to ear during presentation. Thus, brief and relatively meaningless bursts of energy from words or sentences arrive at each ear in a rapid sequence. Lynn and Gilroy (1977) have shown one version of this procedure, which involves sentences, to be particularly sensitive to certain lesions in the low pons and cerebello-pontine angle region of adult subjects. Another sentence version, which is the fourth and final test in the Willeford Battery, has been reported by Miltenberger Caruso, Correia, Love, and et al (1979) to reveal astonishingly poor performance in deep sea divers with decompression sickness (the

Table 25
Binaural Fusion Test Norms* from the Willeford Battery

Age	N	Mean[‡‡] LE – RE	SD[†] LE – RE	Range[†] LE > RE
5	Insufficient at present			
6	40	74.1–75.0	12.2–11.4	55/95 –55/100
7	40	76.0–75.5	12.5–11.9	55/100–55/100
8	40	76.8–76.8	10.3– 8.8	65/100–60/100
9	40	79.9–78.8	11.9–13.2	55/100–55/100
10	40	89.2–87.6	4.8– 5.5	80/95 –75/95
6/10	200	80.6–78.7	10.3–10.2	55/100–55/100

*A correction factor of 10 percent should be added to List 2 scores in the clinical use of the binaural fusion test to balance the relative difficulty of the two lists.
[†]At 30 dB SL.
[‡]Add 5 percent to test norms obtained at 40 dB SL.

"bends"). However, Willeford and Billger (1978), using a 30-dB SL presentation level, have found abnormal results on this test in only a small percentage of the children with CAPD whom they have evaluated. The test is easily administered to children and is a generally enjoyable task for them, but in its present form it is not one of the more sensitive tests for children with CAPD. The test norms, shown in Table 26, suggest that it is an easy test for children. However, failure on this test may eventually provide unique insights into the nature of certain CAPDs in children and lead to more appropriate management strategies.

Table 26
Alternating Speech Test Norms* from the Willeford Battery

Age	N	Mean LE – RE	SD LE – RE	Range LE – RE
5	25	99.2– 99.2	2.6–3.9	90/100– 80/100
6	25	98.3– 98.0	2.2–4.6	90/100– 80/100
7	25	98.3– 99.5	2.2–2.2	90/100– 90/100
8	25	98.8– 99.5	1.4–2.2	90/100– 90/100
9	25	98.8– 99.8	1.4–1.4	90/100– 90/100
10	25	99.8–100.0	1.4–0.0	90/100–100/100
5/10	150	98.9– 99.3	1.9–2.4	90/100– 80/100

*Left and right ears scored according to ear in which stimulus items are initiated (lead ear). Each ear becomes the lead ear 10 times after 20 items—Lists A and B.

Masking Level Differences.   The masking level difference (MLD) procedure is a binaural task that permits the measurement of the release from masking in normal hearing subjects when the test signal (500 Hz pure tones or spondaic words) and its masker (narrowband noise and speech noise, respectively) are presented in and out of phase. A minimal release from masking is thought to reflect low brainstem dysfunction when one's peripheral hearing sensitivity is within normal limits (Olsen, Noffsinger, & Carhart, 1976). It can be easily and quickly administered to children, and Sweetow and Reddell (1978) feel that it holds promise when used as part of a test battery.

ELECTROPHYSIOLOGICAL TESTS

Objective tests that employ electrophysiological protocols have been used to assess central auditory function and have gained popularity over the years. As shown in Table 27, these procedures include aural reflex assessments and measures of auditory evoked potentials in the CANS. Being objective tests, these measures are free of the contaminating influences that may affect subjective (behavioral) tests.

Aural Reflex Test.   The measurement of the crossed and uncrossed reflexes of the stapedial muscle to tonal stimuli is a test of brainstem disorder. It is simple and quick to administer. Jerger (1975) reported that the uncrossed (ipsilateral) reflexes should be present and the crossed (contralateral) reflexes absent when brainstem pathology interferes with the reflex arc (see Figure 22). While various combinations of reflexes resulting from ipsilateral and contralateral stimuli are possible, clinicians should especially take note of the absence of reflexes to contralateral stimulation since it suggests interference with the reflex arc at the lower level of the brainstem. Certainly further diagnostic follow-up to rule out gross pathology is warranted in the event of such findings.

Table 27
Electrophysiological Tests

Aural Reflex—measurement of the crossed and uncrossed reflexes of the stapedial muscle.

Brainstem Evoked Response—measurement of early electrical potentials of the CANS.

Cortical Evoked Response—measurement of late electrical potentials of the CANS.

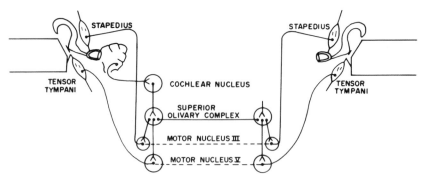

Figure 22. Diagram illustrating the basic components of the crossed and un-crossed neural pathways that make up the acoustic or intra-aural muscle reflex arc. The reflex arc for both the stapedius and tensor tympani are shown; however, at present the stapedius reflex is assumed to make the major contribution to changes measured by impedance instruments (From McCandless G. Impedance measures. In W. Rintelmann (Ed.), *Hearing assessment.* Baltimore: University Park Press, 1979, 281–320. With permission.)

Brainstem Evoked Response. The measurement of brainstem evoked responses (BSER), or early evoked potentials, is another method of objectively measuring processes in the CANS as defined in Table 28. This test has fired the imagination of audiologists and allied professionals. In fact, there have been few, if any, developments in the history of audiology that have generated as much professional excitement. Nonetheless, its present clinical value has been primarily in its use with adults and children with frank neurological deficits and with patients whose peripheral hearing acuity is difficult to assess with standard tests. At present, it has been of limited value in identifying children with more subtle CAPDs. In fact, as mentioned in the section on "Etiological Implications," Shimizu, Brown, Capute, and Mahoney (1981) were unable to demonstrate

Table 28
Classical Categories of Auditory Evoked Responses in the
Central Nervous System

Category	Origin	Wave Form	Latency
Early	Brainstem	Fast (100–2000 Hz)	4–8 Msec
Middle	Primary cortical projection area	Fast (5–100 Hz)	8–50 Msec
Late	Primary cortical projection and secondary association areas	Slow (2–10 Hz)	50–300 Msec

neurophysiological abnormality by BSER in children with carefully defined minimal brain dysfunction, a finding in contrast to that of Sohmer and Student (1978). Children in our own clinical population, whose histories and behavioral test results confirm the presence of a CAPD, routinely show negative BSER results, findings that are in agreement with Worthington (1981). However, in another study, Worthington, Beauchaine, Peters, and Reiland (1981) reported positive BSER results in 30 percent of a population of children with severe developmental and/or language delays.

Protti (1983) recently reported that only 2 of 13 subjects identified by behavioral tests had positive BSER results. She concluded that BSER may not be sensitive to all brainstem disorders, but is probably more appropriate than behavioral tests when relating results to specific sites of lesion within the brainstem. We believe the reason for negative BSER results in CAPD children may lie in the nature of the test stimuli employed, which consist of clicks, filtered clicks, tone pips, and tone bursts. While BSER requires enough stimuli that can be time-locked to permit computer summation, these highly redundant signals may not produce sufficient stress on the CANS to reveal subtle abnormalities. The reader may recall our earlier discussion that emphasized that children with subtle central dysfunctions show normal pure tone audiograms. That is, the simpler the test signal, the less it tells you about children with CAPD. As Brugge (1975) stated, "The (neural) responses to pure tones can be poor predictors of the response to complex stimuli." Moreover, BSER responses merely reflect the auditory mechanism's ability to recognize change in a signal—not its processing functions. A potential strength of BSER is that it remains constant regardless of the organism's state of attention. We may find that future modifications of BSER technology, such as studying latency differences in the brainstem to binaural stimulation (Dobie & Berlin, 1979) will result in more useful diagnostic information in identifying CAPD.

Cortical Evoked Response.   Interest in the late potentials, or cortical evoked response (CER) testing began in the late 1930s (Forbes & Morison, 1938; Loomis, Harver, & Hobart, 1938). Nevertheless, the use of CER presently lacks the precision, reliability, and utility of the brainstem technique. However, investigators have now developed the technology for an exciting technique for comprehensive analysis of evoked potentials of the cortex. The development of brain electrical activity mapping (BEAM) may well be the most versatile tool for assessing dynamic functioning of the cortex (Duffy, 1980). This technique is designed to analyze large volumes of evoked potential information from electrical activity across the scalp during controlled stimulation of the ears. In the future we may be able to identify peculiarities in cortical activity that will lead to greater understanding of the neural functions that underlie CAPD and other CANS disorders.

SUMMARY OF AUDIOLOGICAL EVALUATIONS

With the exception of the evolving brain mapping techniques, the tests presented here are only those measures that are most widely used at present. There are others that, with time and use, may prove to have equal or even better utility. There are limitations to all of the tests discussed but, recognizing their shortcomings, they can be useful in supplying valuable knowledge of dysfunctions in the central auditory nervous system. The authors believe that current tests for CAPD represent a valuable beginning in professional efforts to describe and define auditory processes. We accept that some of these measures will fall into disuse as better tests are developed—tests that will provide improved precision and sensitivity, not to mention convenience and ease of administration. Hopefully, as those developments occur, we will be able to gain greater insights into the complex relationships between audition and speech-language behaviors, academic skills, and numerous other human behaviors.

6

Management of Central Auditory Processing Disorders

Numerous pamphlets, books, and manuals have been written for the purpose of reporting therapy procedures for children with CAPD. Some of the programs also purport to accomplish two other goals: (1) to improve a child's language ability, and (2) to help in the remediation of reading problems (Barr, 1972; Behrmann, undated; Eden, Green & Hansen, 1973; Gillet, 1974; Heasley, 1974; Herr, 1969; Oakland & Williams, 1971; Reagan, 1973; Semel, 1976).

Therapy activities that have been developed include procedures to strengthen environmental localization; sequencing of sounds; memory tasks, such as remembering digits and directions; sound blending; and discrimination of speech in noisy backgrounds. Some of the CAPD therapy programs available to the clinician will be reviewed in the following section.

While some clinicians feel that therapy programs alone will help a child with CAPD, others (Barr, 1972; Rampp, 1980) recommend both therapy techniques and parent-teacher management guidelines to aid the child with CAPD. Willeford and Billger (1978) and Lasky and Cox (1983) advocate compensation strategies that are helpful for these children. If the CAPD child also has academic difficulties, perhaps supplemental tutoring would be indicated. Also, if a language disorder is apparent then language therapy should be implemented.

THERAPY TECHNIQUES

Semel Auditory Processing Program

The Semel Auditory Processing Program (SAPP) was developed in 1976 to help teachers remediate auditory processing disorders that relate to "skills involved in reading, cognition, and communication. . . . " (Semel, 1976). In presenting this program, she states that "Auditory training to awaken the child's potential is directed toward releasing the accumulated store of auditory information and ability that was never properly developed. This type of training is ordinarily accomplished through feeding the brain sequentially-ordered micro-units of auditory configuration patterns" (Semel, 1976). Semel also advocates teaching the child to listen to what he/she hears. Auditory attention is directed to the localization of sounds. The child is shown how to recognize, focus on, discriminate, memorize, categorize, integrate, and synthesize the various patterns of all parts that are essential to the total auditory process.

The primary emphasis of the SAPP seems to involve the identification of target sounds in various words. For example, beginning, intermediate and advanced levels of this program have differences in difficulty, but all concentrate on listening to initial and final consonants, vowels, and blends. Therefore, it appears to be Semel's philosophy that a central auditory processing problem can be treated by working primarily on speech-sound identification. Whether this type of task does, in fact, aid a child with a central auditory processing dysfunction in his or her daily complex auditory environment has not been documented to our knowledge. Furthermore, we question whether children with CAPD, at least those in our population, would profit from such a program. In the milder types of CAPD, of which we see a great number, their problem seems to be poor verbal comprehension that results from impaired input under less than ideal listening conditions.

APT: Auditory Perception Training

Willette, Jackson, and Peckins (1970) are the authors of the Auditory Perception Training (APT) program, which is a remediation plan used to train "essential" auditory processing skills based on progressive levels of attainment. In this program, five basic units of study are presented at three levels of difficulty. The units are: (1) auditory memory; (2) auditory motor; (3)auditory figure-ground; (4) auditory discrimination, and (5) auditory imagery. This program is designed for children in primary and intermediate grade levels.

The APT II therapy plan is an extension of the APT program. The APT II plan was developed to help children improve their ability to listen and follow directions. The units of study are similar to those in the APT program, except for the exclusion of auditory discrimination. This program is suggested as appropriate for the young adolescent student who is not performing at age level.

Auditory Perceptual Training Program

Butler, Hedrick, and Manning developed the Auditory Perceptual Training Program (APT) in 1973 (not to be confused with the Willette,

Jackson, Peckins program in the preceding section). A promotional brochure for this program states that it is applicable primarily to students in grades one to three, or LD students through grade six, "who don't know how to pay attention . . . who are easily distracted by classroom noise . . . who have trouble recognizing voices, hearing differences between sounds, and understanding or remembering what they hear . . . ." This remediation plan is also intended for "children who have learning or reading problems related to inadequate or faulty processing of auditory information." If a child fails the Composite Auditory Perceptual Test (described in Chapter 5), this twice-a-week program is recommended by the authors. This remediation program includes 39 tape-recorded lessons that are divided into four basic units that include exercises such as: (1) Listen for Sounds—selective listening, vigilance, temporal sequencing, speech-sound discrimination, and analysis; (2) Listen for Words and Speakers—intonation patterns, voice identification, temporal sequencing, auditory closure, and auditory synthesis; (3) Listen to Remember—recognition of the number of sounds and syllables in words and phrases and figure-ground discrimination through competing messages, and (4) Listen to Learn—more difficult competing messages and recognition of subject-verb agreement, active and passive voice, and complex syntactical structures. The authors state that, after training with this program, the child will be able to process auditory information more efficiently. Even though the authors state that the program was extensively researched, and was field-tested on over 1500 children, no documentation is provided to support the contention that improvement, if any, is the result of the program rather than of maturation or of other factors.

Auditory Discrimination in Depth Program

The Auditory Discrimination in Depth (ADD) program, developed by Lindamood and Lindamood (1969), was devised "for developing the function of the ear in monitoring the correspondence between the contrasts, sequences, and shifts of our spoken language and the sets of graphic symbols which represent them." The program includes four levels of activities: (1) Gross Level—which includes activities geared to problem-solving techniques and the gross discrimination of sounds; (2) Oral-Aural Level—pertaining to the teaching of auditory discrimination of sounds, consonant/vowel changes in syllable patterns, and changes in syllable combinations; (3) Sound Symbol Level—teaching students to recognize graphic representations for different phonemes, and (4) Coding Level—coding of nonsense syllables into graphic and oral patterns and generalization into works. Finally, a primary goal of this program is to help the child encode and decode multisyllable nonsense patterns until the student has achieved competency with real words (Lindamood & Lindamood, 1969).

The ADD program is recommended as a precursor for any speech, spelling, or reading program and is appropriate for anyone from preschoolers to adults. The length of time that the individual is enrolled in this program varies according to the student's progress. However, the average amount of therapy consists of 40-minute sessions daily for 2–3 months.

Speech-in-Noise Training

Katz and Burge (1971) analyzed the improvement in speech-in-white-noise performance after 8 30-minute therapy sessions with a group of children from 5 to 14 years of age. They noted posttherapy improvement by 2½–3 items in selecting pictorial representations of monosyllabic words presented in the presence of noise. The children could obtain a possible 120–122 correct responses depending upon the test list presented. They averaged 30.9 correct responses on the pretest for monaural presentation of stimuli and 15.1 correct responses by stereo presentation as compared to posttherapy test scores of 34.4 for monaural and 17.6 for stereo listening, respectively.

Trehub (1976), Swoboda, Morse and Leavitt (1976), and Cole (1977) have all suggested that the ability to discriminate speech sounds is an innate talent, and Rees (1973) hypothesizes that if the ability to discriminate speech is innate, perhaps it cannot be improved with therapy. If this is true, it would seem to be equally applicable to speech discrimination in noise.

Phonemic Synthesis Training

Katz and Burge (1971) also studied phonemic synthesis (PS), which is the ability to blend individual phonemes in correct sequence to form a word. Forty-three children from 5–15 years of age enrolled in 8 training sessions of 30 minutes duration. The object was to improve their auditory phonemic synthesis skills. Twenty-nine of these children were used for the final analysis of the success of the program because sufficient test-retest data were not available on all 43 children. The PS therapy program uses prerecorded tapes from which the child is requested to blend two- and three-phoneme words. Seven children were given the Phonemic-Synthesis Multiple Choice Test because of their young age (kindergarten and first grade children) and the severity of their problem. Out of a possible 30 items, the children improved their mean scores of 10.9 correct pretherapy to 25.8 correct posttherapy. The other 22 children were given the Phonemic-Synthesis-2A Test and also demonstrated improvement in their phonemic-synthesis abilities. However, their mean improvement in PS ability was not as great, increasing from a mean score of 10.8 correct to 18.1 correct on the 25 test items for that form.

Katz and Harmon (1981)* report that reasons why PS training might be effective for a child with CAPD include: (1) the child is receiving positive reinforcement from speech improvement; (2) the child develops clearer understanding of speech sounds because the stimuli are clear, prolonged, and repeated; (3) the child learns that words made up of discernable units can be manipulated, and (4) the child now uses his ability to decode new words, which leads to improvement in his reading and spelling ability.

It is interesting to note that Katz and Burge (1971) indicated that the children who showed the greatest improvement in both speech-in-noise and PS skills spanned the age range of five to seven years. The 11- to 12-year-old children exhibited the least amount of improvement using these therapy techniques. The authors felt that the lack of improvement in this age group may have been due to one or more of the following: (1) lowered levels of motivation during therapy; (2) feelings of inadequacy, and (3) this group was beyond the optimum age for developing increased ability in these two skills.

The greatest maturational change in central auditory function occurs in the early years of life—up to age nine or ten as demonstrated by maturational norms of central auditory tests (Berlin et al, 1973; Myrick, 1982; Pinheiro, 1978; Willeford, 1977b; Willeford & Burleigh, see Chapter 5). Perhaps the improvement seen in the younger children in Katz and Burge's study could, in part, be due to maturational development of central auditory function. This may also account for reduced improvement seen among the older children.

The foregoing are only samples of available techniques for aiding children with CAPD. It should be noted that many of these programs were designed to provide the specified therapeutic activities that are thought by some to be important for increasing auditory processing ability, but also to promote associated reading and language skills.

---

*Phonemic Synthesis: Blending Sounds into Words, by Katz and Harmon, is currently available through the Developmental Learning Materials Company, Allen, Texas 75002.

THERAPY AND PARENT-TEACHER MANAGEMENT GUIDELINES

Rampp (1980) has suggested both therapy and parent-teacher management guidelines for the child with CAPD. In general, his program includes therapy in the auditory areas of identification and discrimination, temporal sequencing and memory, and reception. According to the author, these activities are especially appropriate for children from pre-kindergarten to seven years of age. Rampp also provides helpful suggestions for general management as shown in Tables 29 and 30. They include alerting the child verbally to get his or her attention prior to giving instructions, reducing the amount of directions given at one time, giving the child time to grasp information prior to requiring a response, asking specific questions regarding an activity, and speaking clearly and slowly.

For the child over seven years of age, Rampp (1980) recommends specific support in the area of reading and states that the CAPD child will "profit more from a code-emphasis approach . . ." to reading, such as the Initial Teaching Alphabet or the Dystar program.

Some of the same management suggestions for the under-seven age group also apply to older children. Again, instructions should be given using simple language while controlling the complexity of the responses required, i.e., two-part instructions versus five-part instructions. Another management suggestion includes requiring the child to repeat the instructions. This suggestion is designed to gain the child's attention prior to giving directions.

Barr (1972) presents both therapy and classroom management guidelines for CAPD children. He recommends that therapy emphasize aspects of listening such as auditory awareness of sound, localization, rhythm, auditory memory, association, decoding or interpreting meaning from an auditory stimulus, and encoding or the ability to express ideas into words.

Barr not only recommends therapy to aid auditory skills but also suggests methods for controlling auditory input, especially when the child is in the classroom. Some of his suggestions are:

1. Preferential seating should be implemented so that the child can be in optimal visual and auditory locations.
2. The teacher should utilize visual aids when explaining a new concept to the class.
3. Hopefully, the teacher will be alert for signs that the child is not understanding what is being presented to the class.
4. It might be helpful to rephrase material that the child is having difficulty understanding.

Table 29
Parent Suggestions

1. Structure the Environment
   a. Attempt to foster cooperative and understanding relationships in the home. The child needs a stable base.
   b. Provide day-to-day, pleasant learning experiences of a formal or informal nature.
   c. Provide a calm, simple, austere decor.
   d. Use few mirrors and stimulating objects.
   e. Have the workplace facing a blank wall.
   f. Give every child a quiet corner of his own.

2. Punishment
   a. Set consistent limits and standards.
   b. Don't punish a child for behavior that he cannot control, like clumsiness or easy frustration. Spankings are not recommended, for they are often too exciting and violent.
   c. Punishment should be prompt.
   d. Choose appropriate punishment. Don't impose major punishment for a minor transgression.
   e. Avoid long sermons and logical reasonings. Handle the problem directly and simply.
   f. Don't spend excessive time punishing bad behavior at the expense of encouraging good behavior.
   g. Use a child's bed as a place of rest, not as a punishment site.
   h. If you wish to teach a child to hold his temper, then be able to exhibit that behavior yourself.

3. Trouble Prevention
   a. Remove and prevent intolerable stimulation.
   b. Give simple, clear instructions in short series.
   c. When the child exhibits impatience about impending activities, help him by building a step-by-step inner picture. Describe in detail any and all facets of the activity, such as its purpose, any stops, and interesting sights to be expected.
   d. Anxious children can be made more comfortable about expected events if they are predictable as to time, place, etc. Meals should be at regular times, and activities can be scheduled somewhat consistently.
   e. Parents should appear unified on issues to the child, and should avoid disagreement and harsh criticism of each other in front of the child.
   f. Rules of behavior should be definite, simple, and unchanging from parent to parent.
   g. Gradual increases in independence can be achieved by:
      1. Simple, useful, needed household chores.
      2. Encouragement of special talents and interests.

Reprinted from Rampp D. *Auditory processing and learning disabilities.* Omaha, Nebraska: Cliff Notes, 1980, 97–99. With permission.

Table 30

Fourteen Teaching Techniques

The following techniques will be of use to teachers:

1. Group the children in a way that will make it possible to work with them effectively.
2. Teach children in a way that provides maximum feedback on what they are learning and where they are having difficulty.
3. Make use of the feedback.
4. Gear the presentation to the lowest member of the group.
5. Don't be afraid of looking back.
6. Make maximum use of study periods; reduce homework to a minimum. The less control you have, the less you know that the child is learning what he is supposed to learn.
7. Learn to isolate the concepts. This means that the concept must admit to one and only one interpretation—the desired one.
8. Don't use complicated demonstrations; always seek the simplest form in which to present a concept.
9. Don't correct the child by appealing to his intuition or his thinking habits— program rules for thinking.
10. Preserve the child's self-image, but tell him when his answers are wrong.
11. Give the child ample evidence that he is capable of learning.
12. Structure the teaching sessions so that the children work for no more than five to eight minutes on a particular series of tasks.
13. Use fun examples and tasks with a payoff.
14. Concentrate on those aspects of the curriculum that can be accelerated.

Reprinted from Rampp D. *Auditory processing and learning disabilities*. Omaha, Nebraska: Cliff Notes, 1980, 97. With permission.

5. The teacher should speak clearly and use natural gestures if the child is not distracted by them.
6. The teacher should ask short, simple questions, and the child should repeat questions the teacher has asked.
7. Multiple questions or directions should be avoided for this child. Also, it is helpful to isolate key words, so that the child learns to focus on important parts of the auditory signal.
8. An emphasis on phonics should be considered, along with teaching reading by stressing a phonics approach.
9. Discrimination, rhythm, sequencing, and memory activities should be included in the curriculum for this child.

In summary, Barr's approach to management of the child with CAPD is a multi-faceted approach that includes both therapeutic techniques and management suggestions. We feel that both Barr's and Rampp's suggestions in the area of management can be very helpful.

Tallal and her colleagues have provided some possible management insights by exploring the relationships between the processing of speech-like and nonspeech-like auditory stimuli in children with severely delayed language and those with normal language development. Their insights were based in part on an earlier investigation by Tallal and Piercy (1974) in which 12 severely language-delayed children performed poorly when they were asked to identify, discriminate, and sequence auditory stimuli incorporating brief or rapidly changing temporal events. When the duration of the auditory stimuli was increased, the deficits disappeared. Therefore, the longer the duration of the stimulus, the easier it becomes for language-delayed children to process auditory information. Interestingly, Stark and Tallal (1979) also noted that children who have difficulty processing rapidly-changing auditory stimuli often have articulation problems, especially in conversational discourse.

An important observation from these studies is that, even though a child is able to perceive phonemes in isolation, he or she may not be able to effectively discriminate stimuli when they are combined. Moreover, if a child is having difficulty discriminating rapidly-presented phonemes, it may ensue that he or she will have difficulty learning language. An adult can interpret a speech message that is not acoustically pure because they have a better command of language, but a child with CAPD may have difficulty trying to decipher the message, especially when trying to learn new language concepts. Therefore, Tallal and her colleagues stress the importance of pure speech signals. Furthermore, our own clinical experiences have shown that persons with CAPD may have difficulties with phonetic transcriptions and in learning a second language.

Stark and Tallal (1981) recommend that language-training strategies include utilizing the strongest modality for input during therapy and/or teaching the child compensatory skills that especially capitalize on the visual modality. Redundant presentation of new material may be helpful, as may decreasing the number and rate of motor activities required of the child. They further recommend that children seen for language therapy receive complete diagnostic testing, including evaluation of the child's ability to process information visually, auditorially, and motorically. They contend that a child who functions below age level in language skills, and also demonstrates a similar age-level deficiency in visual-spatial and visual-motor skills, should not be classified as specifically language impaired and perhaps should be placed in a different special education program apart from specific language remediation.

COMPENSATION STRATEGIES

In our opinion, research to date has failed to convincingly demonstrate that therapy for CAPD improves a child's auditory skills—at least for practical, everyday listening in complex environments. A child may increase his ability to perform selected listening skills such as phonemic recognition, but an increase in the child's social and academic function, particularly in noisy and active listening environments, has not been documented.

It appears that children with CAPD can be classified into two distinct categories of function. One category involves the child who has a CAPD and also has a language problem. The second category includes the child with a CAPD who does not manifest a language dysfunction but does demonstrate academic and social difficulties. If a child with a CAPD has a language disorder, an appropriate management program should include a comprehensive language therapy program. However, if the child with a CAPD does not have a language problem, a compensatory strategy-management program should be implemented. As alluded to in Chapter 1, there appears to be considerable confusion about the cause-and-effect relationships of CAPDs and language-learning disorders. As we have stated previously, these two phenomena are not unvariable concomitants and can exist as autonomous clinical entities. Therefore, caution should be exercised that CAPD and language-learning disorders not be used interchangeably.

The child with a CAPD who does not manifest a language problem is often discovered because of academic problems and/or social difficulties. This child experiences frustration while trying to handle his everyday environment. He has trouble maintaining the academic pace and in gaining social acceptance. Educationally, these children are often labeled as underachievers, nonachievers, or academic failures. In some cases they become school dropouts. One can readily perceive how frustrating this lack of success would be for the child, his parents, and his teachers. This child demonstrates that he has the native ability to succeed, but the ability to achieve success has eluded him. His social traumas accompany, and are frequently exacerbated by, problems in school.

Ayres (1972) states that the ultimate goal of any sensory therapeutic program is for an individual to react and conduct himself in a meaningful way in response to the requirements of the environment. In other words, children need to develop ways in which they can successfully cope with the demands of their daily environment. Schain (1977) has indicated that the four aspects of the management of any child with a learning disorder include: (1) diagnostic evaluation; (2) parent counseling; (3) educational management, and (4) psychological therapies.

Hopefully, with compensatory management, the child will be able to cope with the various auditory commands placed upon him at home and at school, and consequently be able to break the failure cycle. Inappropriate structure, incomprehensible commands, and tasks that continually lead to failure will not help the child cope with his CAPD. These situations will only result in continued frustration for the child, parents, and teachers. The child must learn to compensate for the auditory disorder and, hopefully, be able to experience success. Management, regardless of type, must be able to help the child to increase his academic and social skills and to improve his self-image as rapidly as possible. This must result from successful experiences which are meaningful to the child.

For the past decade, we have counseled children with CAPD, their families, and appropriate educational personnel regarding ways of helping children to accommodate to the demands of their environments. The suggestions that are shown in Tables 31 and 32 are fundamental and practical guidelines that developed from our own insights and out of our interactions with school personnel, parents, psychologists, and others. In view of the heterogeneity of the population, the guidelines are not equally applicable for each child. Therefore, one must have a good understanding of the child's personality, interests, and auditory difficulties and modify the suggestions accordingly. Flexibility regarding the management of each child is a must for successful implementation of a compensatory approach to this disorder.

SURVEY OF THE EFFECTIVENESS OF COMPENSATION STRATEGIES

In an effort to assess the value of our compensation strategy recommendations, a survey form, shown in Figure 23, was mailed to 100 parents of children with confirmed CAPD. The results of the 67 respondents indicate that, where parents and teachers can and do follow the recommendations provided, the child's performance and self-concept are remarkably improved. In instances where the parents were unable to implement the recommendations at home, or to obtain cooperative efforts from the child's teachers, no changes were effected.

Parents were asked to indicate their feelings about the CAPD evaluation and which compensation-strategy recommendations, if any, they found helpful, and which helped the least. While not all respondents addressed those questions specifically, the following responses do provide some interesting insights.

I feel the tests and recommendations were very helpful. Mostly it taught us to understand what her surroundings are like to her and to understand that, even

Table 31

Compensation Strategies for Teachers of Children with
Central Auditory Processing Disorders

Children with central auditory deficiencies are generally youngsters with normal hearing in the usual sense. That is, they have the sensitivity with which to hear very faint sounds, and they make discriminations between the fine differences (the various phonetic elements) of speech under favorable listening circumstances. However, such children have difficulty "listening to" or "maintaining attention for" speech that is delivered in a complex environment or that is not spoken clearly. They simply cannot use auditory information efficiently.

All competition for the attention of these children should be minimized wherever possible by giving instructions and teaching important concepts where there are the fewest auditory and visual distractions present. Since the processing of complex messages or competing sensory stimuli is very difficult for such youngsters, they perform better when instruction is presented in the simplest terms possible and when you have their undivided attention. This means that, in a controlled or structured auditory environment where distractions are minimal, they will function best when they are in close proximity to you and when you "personalize" that instruction. In other words, stand close to them and use their name frequently to help hold their attention. Seeking periodic feedback from the child also helps to assure that he is following the instruction, and it enhances the child's listening habits since he knows he is expected to "feedback" occasionally. The teacher's speech should also be well articulated, and manners and gestures during the speech act should be subdued so as not to visually distract the child with extraneous movements.

It is desirable to experiment with different seating arrangements for these children. Try seating them in different locations to discover the place where their auditory reception appears best. This position is sometimes unpredictable, but is usually away from doorways, windows facing on the playground, and pencil sharpeners.

Other recommendations that have often proved to be successful for such children are:

1. Reduction of motor activities during the communication process. That is, reduce the number of written responses you require of them.
2. Move into new areas of academic instruction by gradual transition, always reviewing known material first, so that the child can experience some degree of success.
3. Settle for limited successes by praising any accomplishment that represents improvement over previous levels. It is not helpful to demand performance which is comparable with normal children.
4. When the previous suggestions are not possible, repeat instruction to the youngster on an individual basis after class.
5. Use the "buddy" system of having another child assist the one in need.
6. Record lessons or instruction on tape so that the child can hear the material repeated at a later time.

Table 31 (continued)

7. Have the youngster use sound-protection equipment (earplugs, earmuffs) to reduce background noise.
8. Utilize these concepts on the playground, to whatever degree is possible, through the playground supervisor who should stand near the child and make sure that the rules of the game are understood.

All of these ideas have proved to be helpful to children with central auditory disorders. In some instances, and with certain children, they may all apply. In other children, and under differing circumstances, some of the suggestions may prove helpful while others will not. Environmental conditions at home and at school vary widely, so that it may simply not be feasible to implement some of the items mentioned. They are merely recommendations to serve as guidelines and will not apply to all children equally. We know that certain youngsters adapt and compensate with widely ranging skills. Teachers spend a great deal of time with a given child and are perhaps in the best position to determine which techniques are better for him.

We advise the parents about the kinds of activities they can employ at home. You may wish to arrange a conference with the parents to exchange ideas about the approaches that seem to meet with the greatest success for their child. Remember that you, the teacher, can be an extremely influential person in helping the child with an auditory processing problem to progress academically and socially. In so doing, you can give that child a new self-image and restore lost confidence.

---

though she cannot learn all that other children her age can learn, she can be taught to learn as much through other teaching methods. The word-testing with the machines was the most interesting and surprising, as she was having trouble even coming close to the right words. I feel the question and answer period at the end of the evaluation was great, because up to that point I could see she had a problem but didn't know why or how to help her cope with it. Moore School, which she attends, is making a lot of changes next year for children with Diana's problem. I feel your recommendations to the school helped greatly in making them realize that all of these children need special help desperately. Moore is teaching new classes next year for these kids and is getting a few teachers to teach longer sessions with these kids. I think it finally made them realize that she isn't a bad or dumb, lazy kid. Diana appears to be more eager to do things; she seems to be getting brighter and sharper, as if she is progressing more than expected.

Having a valid reason for problems Kristy was having both at home and at school, plus the authority of your institution to back it up. Just the understanding of the problem helped me to change things to make it easier for Kris, i.e., not giving instructions from one room with Kris in another; being patient and restating my question when the response I got did not make sense.

Table 32

Compensation Strategies for Parents of Children with
Central Auditory Processing Disorders

Your child was seen by an audiologist at our hearing clinic and was found to have a central auditory processing disorder. Such children, in spite of having absolutely normal hearing in the usual sense (detecting faint sounds and discriminating between the more subtle sounds of speech), often cannot use sound in an efficient and meaningful manner. They have particular trouble in paying attention to and understanding speech in many of life's situations. For example, these youngsters have considerably more difficulty than other children in listening to speech in any room or environment where the acoustics are poor. They are also at a greater-than-usual disadvantage when attempting to listen to persons who turn away while speaking or who drop their voice noticeably at the end of a sentence. They also have more than average trouble trying to listen in situations in which other noise, and sometimes even movement, is present. Moreover, we have learned that some children are distracted more by events occurring in their visual fields (almost any kind of movement) than they are by background sounds. In many instances, these "other" auditory or visual events seem to interfere, retard, or distort the central nervous system processing rather than distract the child per se. That is, a given child may show little visible recognition of background auditory and visual activities, but central processing nonetheless seems to be interfered with in a very subtle way. The more obvious child, on the other hand, seems to "chase shadows." That is, this type of child actively and overtly shifts his/her attention to other stimuli intruding from the environment. Thus, they can seldom fix their attention on a given task for any length of time.

We have made some suggestions by which your child's teachers can be of greater assistance at school, both in the classroom and on the playground. Following are some guidelines that can be helpful to both you and your child at home. These guidelines are designed to make your child's listening tasks easier. For example, you will have much greater success in communicating with your youngster if there are no other activities (other children or adults laughing or talking, television or radio playing, or the dishwasher or vacuum sweeper running) competing with you. This kind of background noise will seriously interfere with your message, regardless of how hard the child attempts to pay attention. Listening under these conditions is simply more difficult for your youngster than it is for others.

This kind of difficulty means that you must learn to control the environment by obtaining quiet through any means available to you (e.g., take the child to a quiet room, shut off the TV, or ask others to be quiet for a moment). If you can't control the auditory environment immediately, then it would be best to delay your conversation until you can find a quiet time. It would be desirable for you and others in the family to make a point of finding such "quiet conversation periods" on a regular basis during the course of each day. Moreover, it is helpful if you can provide a quiet room in which your child can get away to study and/or play.

Table 32 (continued)

These suggestions are things your child can also learn to employ with the family and with friends. For example, the child can simply learn to avoid important conversations in noisy places, moving the speaker to a quieter environment, getting the speaker on the side of his "strong" ear (this is important for seating arrangements at school and in auditoriums) and standing close to the speaker.

When talking with your child, it is advisable to use simple language. For example, don't use long words when short words will do. Also, use short sentences that contain only one major idea. You should also pronounce your words carefully. Communication will be easier when you have the child's full attention. Thus, do not try to have discussions when you are in separate rooms or when he is preoccupied with other thoughts and activities. You can also help your child by setting firm controls in daily living activities. Structure all activities so that the child has fewer opportunities to be confused. The formation of daily routines and schedules will help him/her to achieve some measure of success—something every child needs to maintain self-esteem. Minor successes (anything that presents an improvement, even though the performance is below normal standards) are small landmarks of growth and maturity which you can legitimately reward. These recommendations are often particularly applicable to the child's poor time perceptions, that is, a seeming lack of concern for punctuality and starting and finishing tasks on schedule.

A final word. These children, like all other children, also need discipline. However, they should always know what behavior is being punished and why. You should also be certain, whenever possible, that you avoid punishing behavior that the child could not help. Thus, it is important that you set enforceable rules for the child to live by.

In summary, you can simplify your child's auditory task by conducting your conversation in the same room, standing close, making sure you have the youngster's undivided attention, using clear and simple language, and trying to minimize all other noise and movement activity. Routine living patterns and enforceable rules can also be helpful.

There are other suggestions that we hope to be able to pass along to you as we learn more about this problem. In the meantime, please call or write our clinic if any particular problem arises on which you feel the need for assistance.

All very helpful. We were most happy with your explanation to Anita regarding her difficulty, and in explaining various methods to her in helping her to control how to make the best use of incoming information.

Touching Cindy and talking directly to her. At first not giving her so many tasks or directions at once. Factors that affect her listening ability still and are often uncontrollable are fatigue and new people visiting. She will "accommodate" by escaping from listening—pretends not to be interested when I think it is a time when she doesn't have the strength to work at listening. Instructions on how to talk directly to Cindy. Awareness of difficult listening situations and how to make them easier for Cindy.

Always speak to his face and make sure he is watching me. I find most of my problems start when I don't do this. Also, his classwork fails when his teacher doesn't make sure he understood.

Awareness that background noises are distracting. I liked having *written* suggestions that I could re-read and share with others (teachers at school, church, etc.).

The staffing at Fort Collins High was the turning point for Bob. The staffing was very productive and informative in that there was a representative of all interested parties (CSU, high school, school district, and parents). Up to this point Bob hated school, was cutting classes and just didn't care. Now he likes school and is a little impatient for it to start again.

Actually changing the total school environment helped the most—understanding that stimuli could and should be controlled—reducing distractions and a focused academic program seems to be the key to confidence and progress for Joe.

Explaining her problem to her and explaining how she could compensate for it. She has gained a lot of self-confidence. Also, her position in the classroom was changed and the earmuffs made it possible for her to concentrate better. At first she didn't want to wear the earmuffs, but after the teacher in the resource room let more of them out for use, she wasn't so self-conscious. Everyone at the center is always helpful. I really enjoy the experience. I do wish there were workshops for more teachers to understand this problem and help all the kids who have it.

Repeating instructions in a positive manner because we understood when he didn't follow through that it was because he didn't understand, *not* that he was disregarding instructions.

They all helped the most—getting earplugs—knowing she has the difficulty so we and the teacher can change habits to suit her needs.

At this time she is in the fourth grade and in a much more controlled atmosphere at school. At home, we now realize what Dynee's special needs are and how to deal with them. It has surely made her life much better and happier, as well as ours. She also has a great teacher who works well with her and understands all of her needs and meets them well. The tests and recommendations which you have offered have been a great help to us. I really believe that without your help and insight, this child could have been seriously abused.

In the final analysis, offering recommendations for compensatory behaviors and environmental modifications represents an important step in the management of children with CAPD. It immediately addresses the fundamental problems of the child and offers many children the oppor-

Management Survey and Responses from 67 Parents.
COLORADO STATE UNIVERSITY
Fort Collins, CO 80523

To:

Re:

Dear

In an effort to learn more about the nature of central auditory disorders, we would appreciate your taking the time to complete and return this brief questionnaire about your child whom we evaluated at our clinic. Check any and all items that seem appropriate, and please add comments if you think they will be helpful in guiding our future efforts to understand this apparently widespread problem.

A. Changes that have occurred at school as the result of our recommendations:
- 11* 1. There has not been adequate opportunity to try them.
- 11 2. Little interest has been shown by the teachers.
- 43 3. The teachers have been helpful and cooperative.
- 27 4. Our child's seating arrangement has been changed.
- 25 5. Our child has been placed in a resource room for certain periods of instruction.
- 29 6. Our child is now receiving more individual attention and assistance.
- 11 7. Other_____

B. Has your child experienced any changes?
- 34 1. Has become more confident.
- 34 2. Is showing fewer frustrations.
- 22 3. Is attempting to control the environment in a productive way.
- 16 4. We have not noticed any change.
- 5 5. Other_____

C. What have your experiences been like?
- 57 1. Relief at having identified a source of some problems.
- 8 2. We are having difficulty in following the recommendations because:
  - 1 a. We don't understand what we are supposed to do.
  - 4 b. We don't know if we are doing the right thing.
  - 3 c. Other_____
- 44 3. We are finding the recommendations helpful.
- 20 4. We feel the need for further counseling.
- 6 5. Nothing has changed.
- 7 6. Other_____

D. Which recommendations helped the most, if any?

E. Which helped the least?

*Number of responses.

Figure 23. Management survey and responses from 67 parents.

tunity to experience some measure of success, which can be supplemented with long-range training procedures that may prove helpful. It affords a large step toward restoring the child's self-confidence and helps him to recapture some measure of academic respectability and social acceptance. These are often the major reasons why these children are brought to our hearing clinic. They had those needs that were not being met.

SOUND-CONTROL DEVICES
(EARMUFFS AND EARPLUGS)

Personal sound-attenuating devices such as earplugs and earmuffs have been employed as treatment for children with CAPD (Hasbrouck, 1980; Willeford, 1980a; Willeford & Billger, 1978). Such an approach can be rationalized by the common knowledge that shows that individuals with an impaired CANS tend to have significant difficulty processing auditory information in unfavorable acoustic environments. Thus, by occluding the weak ear and, therefore, improving the conditions under which auditory signals arrive, a reduction in stress is placed on the impaired system, which allows for better comprehension of the message. The figure-ground, or signal-to-noise ratio, is also enhanced, of course, by strategic seating in the classroom or any auditory environment that will place the child in closer proximity to the desired auditory signal—the speaker, and/or away from sources of auditory competition.

The authors began using such devices on an experimental basis several years ago, based on the knowledge that background sound was a problem for children with CAPD and that it could be suppressed by ear-occlusion devices. Reports from teachers were encouraging from the beginning. Children who were diagnosed as having CAPD were counseled in the selective-use of plugs and/or muffs, that is, to use them in situations where ambient noise interfered with important academic tasks, combine their use with favorable seating arrangements, and use them only when the situation necessitated an advantage. Bilateral occlusion was recommended during desk activities when concentration was important.

Hasbrouck (1980) conducted an ear-occlusion study on 21 LD students who were identified as having figure-ground disorders on the basis of scoring below the 25th percentile on the Noise Subtest of the Goldman-Fristoe-Woodcock (GFW) Test of Auditory Discrimination (1970). He compared the subjects' scores on three randomized versions of the noise subtest while occluding their left ears, right ears, and both ears. Subjects performed better in quiet than in all noise conditions and performed better in the noise conditions while wearing occlusion devices. Eighteen of the 21 subjects improved to greater than the 25th percentile, and 16 did so with unilateral ear occlusion. On the basis of group data, Hasbrouck (1981) subsequently recommended the following treatment procedures:

1. If unilateral ear occlusion improves performance in background noise (on the GFW Noise Subtest), have the patient wear a plug in the ear which produces the best results whenever they must attend to relevant auditory stimuli in noise environments.
2. When performance on the GFW Noise Subtest is superior while wearing bilateral occlusion, have the patient wear plugs in both ears when the background noise is distractable, but when foreground sound is not relevant to the listener.

Reports from parents of children evaluated in our clinic suggest that plugging does have practical value. In addition, school personnel have found occlusion devices useful. This is particularly true when the child is working individually at his desk and wants to eliminate classroom noise in order to concentrate on his assignments (Willeford & Billger, 1978). Obviously, the use of bilateral occlusion devices is not indicated during periods of oral instruction by the teacher.

Because we had no solid data, we conducted a survey of 81 families with children having confirmed CAPD and to whom we had supplied plugs for experimental use. Our interest was to determine how many children were helped by the plugs, in what environmental conditions they were found useful, and whether they were more effective when worn in the weak ear or strong ear as determined by central auditory test performance. Although we continue to recommend that the children experiment with plugs in the weak ear and the strong ear, greater satisfaction has been reported when the weak ear is occluded.

A possible explanation for improved figure-ground listening by blocking sound to the weak ear might be the reduction of neurological interference from the weak ear to the strong ear, even though Speaks (1975) has shown that such occurs with CVs but not with SSI sentences. One could argue that there is no apparent logic to plugging the strong ear since that would place greater dependence on the weak ear. In real life situations, the listener would logically utilize environmental positioning with combinations of body and head movements to achieve figure-ground advantages. It seems reasonable to believe that listeners with a unilateral weakness would wish to compensate for maneuvering their unoccluded strong ear toward the primary message. Furthermore, if the weaker ear does contaminate bilateral integration skills, blocking sound to the weak ear with plugs would eliminate or reduce the possibility of such contamination.

To make the unilateral occlusion decisions based on group data, or on static listening tests conducted in a sound-field, seems inappropriate. To do so would not help to define unilateral and bilateral strengths of the CANS. However, CAP tests used to establish the relative strengths of the two ears are helpful in making decisions regarding the implementation of unilateral occlusion.

DRUG THERAPY

The use of psychoactive drugs as treatment for children with learning problems has had a controversial history. This is probably a natural consequence of reports that range from dramatic improvements in behavior or performance to undesirable side-effects, such as drowsiness and withdrawal, and no change in primary goal behaviors. We have had reports from parents of children who were evaluated for CAPD both praising and criticizing the use of drugs. The major value, when observed, is the calming effect they have on "hyperactive" children who become management problems. However, other parents prefer to live with hyperkinetic behavior rather than the alternative, which one mother described as turning her son into a "good little zombie." There are also a substantial number of parents who are staunch opponents of drug therapy under any circumstances. When drugs work, they represent a "quick remedy." The child slows down, shows better attention, less distractability and, on occasion, demonstrates improved cognitive skills and academic performance. For other children, little change in behavior is noted, or hyperactivity is slowed but improvement is not observed in the child's classroom performance. Certainly, drugs are not a panacea, particularly when educational gains are negligible (Aman, 1980) and when certain behavioral interventions achieve more favorable results (Gadow, 1983).

Two important factors make it difficult to assess the relative effects of drugs in the treatment of behavior and learning problems. First, the type of drug is important since some drugs are stimulants which are intended to increase productivity, whereas antidepressant drugs are generally given to control social behavior, attention span, and emotion. Second, some children are also known to react quite differently from others to a given medication and may well be influenced by variations in dosage and duration of the treatment period.

Sprague and Sleator (1976) demonstrate the interaction of dosage and response in Figure 24, which shows that a dosage sufficient to control social behavior reduces cognitive performance. Conversely, the dosage that maximizes cognitive performance is too little to bring undesirable

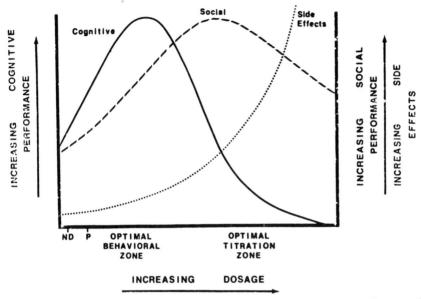

Figure 24. Theoretical dose-response curves (Sprague R, & Sleator E. Drugs and dosages: Implications for learning disabilities. In R Knights & D Bakker (Eds.), *The neuropsychology of learning disorders.* Baltimore: University Park Press, 1976, 351–366. With permission.

social behaviors under control. In the latter case, the elimination of antisocial behaviors may represent over-control by virtue of the undesirable side-effects shown by Schain (1977) in Table 33 for four commonly used drugs. An excellent review of the relative benefits of drugs on LD children has been presented by Aman (1980) and is summarized in Tables 34 and 35. His conclusion, based on a wide range of studies, is that there is little compelling evidence to support the fact that psychotropic drugs have value for achieving educational gains. An even more current update on the effectiveness of drugs in ameliorating learning and behavior problems in children is provided in the review and discussion of issues by Gadow (1983). He concludes that there is some evidence that academic productivity may be increased by stimulant drugs in some hyperactive children, but that such gains are not impressive and that they have little carryover to adolescent and adult years. Moreover, the minimal gains noted are generally confined to relatively unimportant school activities. Dimond (1976) has suggested that "it may be that an ounce of a drug rather than the collected weight of libraries of theoretical speculation will prove itself the most effective agent for therapy for learning disorders." However, the literature reviews by both Gadow and Aman support the

Table 33

Dosage Levels of Drugs Used in Treatment of Hyperactivity

Drug	Range of Daily Dosage	Important Side Effects
Methylphenidate (Ritalin)	5–40 mg (0.3–1 mg/kg)	Personality changes Withdrawal
Dextroamphetamine (Dexedrine)	5–20 mg (0.2–0.5 mg/kg)	Personality changes Withdrawal
Thioridazine (Mellaril)	20–60 mg (0.5–1 mg/kg)	Drowsiness, dystonia, jaundice (rarely), leukopenia, rash
Imipramine (Tofranil)	10–150 mg	Personality changes, drowsiness, hypertension (Werry et al, 1975)

Reprinted from Schain R. *Neurology of childhood disorders* (ed 2). Baltimore: Williams & Wilkins, 1977, 137.

notion that drugs represent a questionable alternative for assisting LD children. Moreover, these reviewers concur that objective knowledge on the subject is difficult to obtain because of the numerous variables that can contaminate research outcomes.

Perhaps an overriding factor in the continued use of, and research in, behavior-modifying medications is the social and ethical considerations. Schain (1977) presents a comprehensive discussion of issues that should be considered by the prescribing physician, other professionals, and parents before placing children on drug programs. He warns physicians of their responsibility when engaging in the practice of personality alteration through pharmacology, which he feels obviates the promotion of self-control by the child and has profound consequences for subsequent personality and cognitive development. Moreover, Schain cautions that continuation of drugs for more than several months may lead to subtle dependence on such medications. The use of drugs, and the accurate reporting of the child's response to them, is another concern he expresses since drug abuses may impede future benefits that might accrue by positive parental and professional management. Perhaps it is fortunate that notable abuses are reported by the lay media. One particular case serves as a noteworthy example. A group of parents in the Taft (California) City School District filed and won a class action lawsuit against the District to halt the practice of coercing children into taking methylphenidate (ritalin) as a condition for attending public school (Bell, 1980). The problem was brought into focus when it was discovered that a surprisingly large number of the children on ritalin were suffering from loss of

Table 34

Drug Studies in Children with Learning Problems

Researchers	Subjects	Drug and Dose	Results	
Conners, Rothschild, Eisenberg, Schwartz, & Robinson, 1969	Learning disability, further unspecified	Dextroamphetamine (25 mg/day)	Reading	NS*
			Arithmetic	.05*
Conrad, Dworkin, Shai, & Tobiessen, 1971	Hyperactive; extent of educational retardation not indicated.	Dextroamphetamine (10 to 20 mg/day)	Reading	NS†
			Arithmetic	NS*
Conners, Taylor, Meo, Kurtz, & Fournier, 1972	Minimal brain dysfunction; extent of backwardness unspecified	Dextroamphetamine (20 mg/day)	Reading	.05*
			Reading	NS*
			Arithmetic	NS*
Rie, Rie, Stewart, & Ambuel, 1976a	Backward in reading by at least 6 months	Methylphenidate (X = 21 mg/day)	Reading	NS*
			Arithmetic	NS*
Rie, Rie, Stewart, & Ambuel, 1976b	Backward in reading by at least 6 months	Methylphenidate (X = 23 mg/day)	Reading	NS*
Gittelman-Klein & Klein, 1976	Backward in reading by at least 2 years	Methylphenidate (X = 53 mg/day)	Reading (4 weeks)	NS*
			Reading (12 weeks)	NS*
		Methylphenidate	Arithmetic (4 wks)	.001*
			Arithmetic (12 wks)	NS*
Arman & Werry (in press)	Reading retarded. Mean reading deficit of 3.6 years relative to mental age	Methylphenidate (0.35 mg/kg/day) Diazepam (0.1 mg/kg/day)	Reading	NS*
			Psycholinguistic Assessments	NS*

Adapted from Aman M. Psychotropic drugs and learning problems—9 selective review. *Journal of Learning Disabilities*, 1980, 13(12), 36–46.
*Drug improvement.
†Worsening with drugs.
NS = Not significant.

Table 35
Summary of Follow-up Studies on Education Learning Measures (all studies of hyperactive children)

Authors	Time span	Drugs and group composition	Comparison	Results
Mendelson, Johnson, Stewart 1971	2 to 5 years	83 patients, 92% of whom treated with methylphenidate or dextroamphetamine	Same group over time; no control group	only 65% attending regular schools; 25% in special schools or classes; 58% failed one or more grades at follow-up; 57% had "reading difficulty."
Weiss, Minde, Werry, Douglas, Nemeth 1971	5 years	64 children initially treated with chlor-promazine (also dextroamphetamine, methylphenidate and thioridazine)	37 'matched' normal controls	Hyperactive children worse than controls in oral reading, arithmetic, and writing (school reports). 70% had failed at least one grade in comparison to 15% for controls
			Same group over time	When same group was compared over time, hyperactives performed neither better nor worse. Improvement in verbal IQ (WISC)* over time
Minde, Weiss, Mendelson 1972	5 years	63% of 91 children had initially received phenothiazines; 37% had received dextroamphetamine	Same group over time	No changes in WISC, Goodenough,* or Bender over time.

144

Quinn & Rapoport 1975	1 year	Methylphenidate, $N = 23$ imipramine, $N = 13$	Unmedicated hyperactive children, $N = 12$	WISC, WRAT,* and Porteus Mazes did *not* differ at baseline or at 1 year
Weiss, Kruger, Danielson, Elman 1975	5 years	Methylphenidate, $N = 24$ chlorpromazine, $N = 22$	Unmedicated hyperactive children, $N = 20$, matched for age, sex, IQ, SES	No group differences on WISC, Bender Gestalt,* Goodenough.* No differences on number passing each school grade; tendency for unmedicated group to be less successful in passing grades. WISC verbal score improved for chlorpromazine group over time.
Hechtman, Weiss, Finkelstein, Werner, Benn 1976	10 years	35 children, treatment not stated	25 controls matched for sex, IQ, SES	More hyperactive children expelled from school; tendency for lower academic standing and fewer grades completed.
Riddle & Rapoport 1976	2 years	Methylphenidate, $N = 40$ imipramine, $N = 7$	57 normal boys	Hyperactive children worse than controls on WRAT, arithmetic, and reading.
			Same group over time	Hyperactives lost ground in arithmetic.

Reprinted from Aman M. Psychotropic drugs and learning problems—9 selective review. *Journal of Learning Disabilities*, 1980, 13(12), 36–46. With permission.

*WISC = Wechsler Intelligence Scale for Children, WRAT = Wide Range Achievement Test, Bender Gestalt = Bender Visual-Motor Gestalt Test, Goodenough = Goodenough-Harris Draw A Person Test.

appetite and weight, leg cramps, nightmares, and bed wetting. Press reports such as this underscore Schain's admonition. Audiologists and other professionals need to share in the responsibility of drug therapy by being apprised of the literature, by knowing which children are on psychoactive drugs, and by helping parents, teachers, and others to monitor and report to the prescribing physician the children's responses to drug treatment. This responsibility rests heavily on all involved participants, and particularly on audiologists since many hyperactive and LD children examined for CAPD are on, have been on, or are being considered for, drug therapy. However, the precise effect that such drugs have on central auditory functions per se remains to be established. In the final analysis, drug therapy should not be viewed as the primary management approach for children with CAPD.

DIET CONTROL

Although it lacks the risk of the harmful side-effects associated with drugs, diet control for treating LD and hyperactive children, some of whom may also have CAPD, has been a controversial treatment method. Opposition to special diets by some in the scientific community may not be easy to understand, except that early claims of behavior modification by special additive-free (e.g., coloring and preservatives) diets were largely anecdotal in nature. Also, of course, such claims are poorly received by food manufacturers who incorporate additives in their products. Numerous studies have been conducted to evaluate the merits of the Feingold Diet (an elimination of artificial colorings, artificial flavorings, and natural salicylates from one's diet), but there has been no consensus of this diet's value in terms of hard scientific data. However, some professionals believe that the large number of variables involved, together with methodological differences, preclude objective judgments of the true value of diet therapy. For the interested reader, the June/July 1983 issue of the *Journal of Learning Disabilities* has a series of articles that debate the relative merits of the Feingold Diet. There are a number of parents who have their children follow the Feingold Diet. Mattes (1983) claims that improvement seems more often due to the placebo effect of focusing parental attention on the child's needs than to the diet itself. That is, it helps to get the child the kinds of personal attention that will assist him. At present, we are unaware of evidence that would suggest that dietary controls influence the performance of children with CAPD. Research is needed before we can make an intelligent determination of the value of dietary factors in CAPD children.

7

Central Auditory Processing Disorders: Special Populations

Comparatively little attention has been focused on the impact of CAPD on populations other than those with learning and/or language disorders. However, clinicians need to be aware of the possibility that children with other problems may also have a CAPD. This chapter addresses some of those special populations.

CENTRAL AUDITORY PROCESSING DISORDERS IN CHILDREN WITH OTITIS MEDIA

One of the more interesting issues in recent years has been the influence of otitis media (OM) on central auditory function and learning behaviors in children. This issue has resulted in the generation of controversial literature that has served as the motivation for continuing research. Observations by a broad spectrum of professionals reveal that children with communication and learning problems frequently have histories of middle-ear infections. However, Ventry (1980) believes one should exercise caution when drawing a conclusion about a cause-and-effect relationship. He notes that, while the majority of studies show that OM children typically show inferior performance on the criterion measures employed when compared with non-OM children, selection factors for choosing OM subjects have been almost routinely subjected to criticism. For example, the age of occurrence, the number of episodes, their severity and duration, and the currency and nature of medical management have all been variables that have differed considerably.

The criterion measures themselves have also created semantic confusions. Writers use similar terms to describe different behaviors or to mean different things. That is particularly true for the many measures used to assess auditory and/or language skills. As discussed in Chapter 1, the term "auditory processing" means different things to different professionals. Persons presuming to measure or quantify central auditory processing ability often use tests in which certain theoretical acoustic factors are believed to facilitate given linguistic events. Such tests generally lack validation of that relationship, and the acoustical controls that are normally a fundamental feature of auditory tests are commonly neglected. That is, an auditory processing test is not necessarily an auditory processing test simply because the test stimulus is verbal, since one cannot isolate and confirm the auditory contribution versus the linguistic contribution. The authors believe the test stimulus must be controlled and should uniquely stress the CANS in some way, as stated earlier, while minimizing the role of linguistic content. Thus, emphasis is placed on sampling the integrity of the CANS. The reader will recall that persons with CAPD typically demonstrate normal performance on traditional tests of speech audiometry and function normally in favorable listening environments but have markedly reduced performance when listening tasks are made stressful.

Because such a wide variety of tests have been employed to evaluate the influences of OM, it is not appropriate to compare the results of the numerous studies. Moreover, such studies report group data, which obscures individual performance in the OM group. Although clinical populations (OM, LD, and language-disordered) typically show inferior performances when compared with control subjects, it is not uncommon for certain subjects in those clinical groups to perform better than some controls. In other words, there are wide ranges of performance in all groups on most tests that seek to place stress on the CANS.

The National Institute of Neurological and Communicative Disorders and Stroke (1981) reports that over 50 percent of all children will incur middle-ear infections and that evidence of having had such experience has been shown in 20 percent of school children. Thus, it is not surprising to find considerable evidence of OM in specific clinical populations. Two studies in which diagnostic classifications were controlled found the presence of OM was not more prevalent in children who had CAPD. Burleigh, Skinner and Norris (1982) found that 58 of 188 children with abnormal performance on the Willeford Central Auditory Test Battery had long histories of OM. Conversely, 130 of 188 children with confirmed CAPD did not have histories of OM. In the other study, Young (1983) studied the prevalence of OM in 75 children with confirmed CAPD. All subjects had obtained abnormal scores on Katz' SSW test and the Competing-Sentence and Filtered-Speech tests of the Willeford Battery. She found that 37 out of 75 children had positive histories of OM.

Interesting results have also been observed in the authors' own clinical population. In a random sample of 150 children with CAPD, as assessed with a wide range of CAP tests, 72 had histories of OM. Conversely, the remaining 78 subjects had negative OM histories. Thus, the precise cause-and-effect relationship remains unresolved in our judgment and needs further study. Reviews of conductive hearing loss and its influence on CANS functions may be found in Katz (1978b), Ventry (1980), Webster (1983), and Reichman and Healey (1983).

CENTRAL AUDITORY PROCESSING DISORDERS IN EMOTIONALLY DISTURBED TEENAGERS

According to Chandler and Jones (1983), emotionally disturbed (ED) children are routinely diagnosed as learning disabled (LD) and placed in school programs designed for LD children. The reasons they cite for this course of action include economic, administrative, pedagogical, social, and legal considerations. The problem, they feel, begins with diagnosis. Specifically, what diagnostic criteria are used to determine when a child is ED? They point out that school systems follow the federal definition found in P.L. 94-142, which reads:

> Serious emotional disturbance is a condition exhibiting one or more of the following characteristics, over a long period of time and to a marked degree, which adversely affects educational performance: an inability to learn which cannot be explained by intellectual, sensory, or health factors; an inability to build or maintain satisfactory interpersonal relationships with peers and teachers; inappropriate types of behavior or feelings under normal circumstances; a general pervasive mood of unhappiness or depression; or a tendency to develop physical symptoms or fears associated with personal or school problems. The term includes children who are schizophrenic or autistic [since moved to "Other Health Impaired" category]. It does not include children who are socially maladjusted unless it is determined that they are seriously emotionally disturbed (PL 94-142, REGULATIONS, 1977, Sec. (121a5)).

However, many psychiatrists and psychologists use other formalized definitions.

Chandler and Jones stress that ED does not have an "objective reality" such as mental retardation and, therefore, we make ED whatever we choose to make it. Regardless of which definitions one adopts, the CAP status of individuals who have been classified as ED by psychiatric and psychological sources had not been established until Glasier's study in 1981. She compared the central auditory function of a group of institutionalized teenagers with those of non-ED control subjects who were attending regular high schools. Both groups were given Katz' SSW,

Willeford's Competing Sentence (CS) test, and the Token Test* (DeRenzi & Vignola, 1962). Glasier modified the presentation format of the Token Test by recording the test items on tape and presenting two versions of the stimuli at specified sensation levels. One version had a binaural format in which the signal was presented to both ears under earphones at 50 dB SL. The other version, which was termed the "altered" form, presented test stimuli at 35 dB SL while competing speech-noise was presented to the contralateral ear at 50 dB SL. The results showed that the ED subjects' performance was inferior to that of the controls on all tests. However, it should be noted that the altered version of the Token Test was a more sensitive measure than the binaural format although both tests "appeared to reflect deficits in linguistic competence." Left ears showed poorer performances on all tests for the ED subjects as a group. A seeming limitation to the study was the fact that all of the ED subjects were referred because of suspected CAPD. Thus, the ED subjects may have represented a selective population. It would be most interesting to compare the Ed population in this study with a group of ED subjects in whom CAP problems were not suspected. Glasier and her colleagues are presently conducting a series of studies in which they are assessing a variety of auditory and language parameters in ED adolescents.

CENTRAL AUDITORY PROCESSING DISORDERS IN JUVENILE DELINQUENTS

The prevalence of learning disorders (LD) reported among juvenile delinquents (JD) is alarmingly high, with estimates ranging from 30 percent (Berman, 1976) to as high as 94 percent (Dzick, 1967). Studies of the causes of specific LD in JD populations have been concerned primarily with visual perceptual problems. Such studies have been summarized by Berman and Siegal (1976), Slavin (1978), and others. Studies have also investigated the prevalence of biochemical disorders, neuro-allergies, alcoholism, nutritional deficiencies, and radiation damage in JDs. However, these studies primarily focus on the potential causes of criminal behavior rather than possible reasons for LD. Auditory and/or language deficiencies have received relatively less attention.

---

*The Token Test was originally developed to assess subtle receptive language deficits in aphasic adults. However, McNeil and Prescott (1978) suggest that their revised version of the Token Test is a measure of central auditory function even though the test format was not substantially altered. The auditory presentation of test items is not controlled in either form, a factor that is important for any auditory test. The test involves having the subjects follow verbal commands to manipulate colored geometric symbols.

In an attempt to define the central auditory function of JDs, Smock (1982) administered a series of audiological CAP tests to a group of 30 JD teenagers who were randomly selected from institutionalized subjects at a residential school for youthful offenders in Colorado. Their performance was then compared with that of a matched age-group of non-JDs. Subjects' ages for both groups ranged from 15.2 to 19.0 years, with IQs ranging from 80 to 120. The test battery consisted of three measures from the Willeford Central Auditory Test Battery (Filtered Speech, Binaural Fusion, and Alternating Speech), the Compressed WIPI Test (Beasley & Freeman, 1977), and the Dichotic Digit Test (Musiek et al, 1980). All tests were recorded on magnetic tape, played through tape decks connected to calibrated audiometers, and administered under earphones in sound-controlled test suites.

The results shown in Tables 36 and 37 reflect the number and percent of abnormal CAP scores obtained by the population of JD subjects on each

Table 36
Number and percent* of 30 juvenile delinquent subjects
with abnormal[†] scores on a battery of 5 CAP tests

Tests				
Filtered Speech	Binaural Fusion	Alternating Speech	Compressed Speech	Dichotic Digits
15 (50%)	8 (27%)	16 (53%)	11 (36%)	2 (7%)

Adapted from Smock S. Central auditory skills in juvenile delinquents. Masters thesis, Colorado State University, 1982.
*Percent rounded to the nearest whole number.
[†]Abnormality criterion: Scores which fell below the range of scores obtained by control group of non-delinquent subjects.

Table 37
Number and percent* of abnormal[†] scores by left and
right ears of 30 juvenile delinquent subjects on a battery
of 5 CAP tests

	Tests				
	Filtered Speech	Binaural Fusion	Alternating Speech	Compressed Speech	Dichotic Digits
RE	15 (50%)	7 (23%)	15 (50%)	10 (33%)	1 (3%)
LE	6 (20%)	3 (10%)	7 (23%)	5 (17%)	1 (3%)

Adapted from Smock S. Central auditory skills in juvenile delinquents. Masters thesis, Colorado State University, 1982.
*Percent rounded to the nearest whole number.
[†]Abnormality criterion: Scores which fell below the range of scores obtained by control group of non-delinquent subjects.

of the CAP tests. The criterion for judging abnormality was any score that fell below the range of scores (below the poorest normal scores on each test) obtained by the control group. Even by this stringent criterion, the evidence suggests that JDs, as a group, have poor central auditory functions. That evidence is even more dramatic when viewed in the manner shown in Table 38, which is the number of failed responses by one ear compared with both ears. These data reveal that 14 of the 30 JDs failed some test in the battery in both ears and that 29 of the 30 subjects had an abnormal performance on one of the tests in at least one ear. Stated differently, 97 percent of the JDs showed diagnostic evidence of a CAP dysfunction on this particular test battery. These results would seem to confirm: (1) the value of test batteries as opposed to a single measure of central auditory function, and (2) a high incidence of central auditory deficiency among JDs. Such results lead one to wonder to what degree, if any, that deficits in central auditory function might play in the concurrence of JD.

Smock (1982) noted that her subjects evidenced poor academic performance during their elementary school years that, according to most of the case histories, was associated with behavior problems of some sort. Their teachers characterized approximately 50 percent of the JDs as daydreamers, slow starters, poor listeners, impulsive, frustrated, and with short attention spans and the tendency to give up easily. As stated in Chapter 3, the authors believe that each of these behaviors, and others, may be directly linked to CAPD.

Table 38
Number and percent* of abnormal[†] scores by one or
both ears of 30 juvenile-delinquent subjects on a battery
of 5 CAP tests

	Tests				
	Filtered Speech	Binaural Fusion	Alternating Speech	Compressed Speech	Dichotic Digits
One Ear	9 (30%)	7 (20%)	10 (33%)	7 (23%)	2 (7%)
Both Ears	6 (20%)	2 (7%)	6 (20%)	4 (13%)	0 (0%)

Adapted from Smock S. Central auditory skills in juvenile delinquents. Masters thesis, Colorado State University, 1982.
*Percent rounded to the nearest whole number.
[†]Abnormality criterion: Scores which fell below the range of scores obtained by control group of non-delinquent subjects.

CENTRAL AUDITORY PROCESSING IN
THE HEARING-AID USER

For years, audiologists have used peripheral hearing test results to help determine optimal hearing aid fitting for both adults and children. Typically, a comprehensive diagnostic battery is comprised of air and bone conduction tests, speech audiometry via earphones and sound field, comfortable loudness levels, tolerance testing, and impedance audiometry. Tests for assessing the integrity of the CANS have typically not been employed prior to hearing aid fitting. When one considers that the majority of our listening time is spent in complex listening environments that tax the CANS instead of in perfectly quiet situations, the rationale for assessing one's ability to handle complex auditory information prior to hearing aid selection is extremely strong.

In the past, audiologists have been concerned with evaluating central auditory function for site-of-lesion purposes, but more recently attention has been directed toward evaluating the CANS to determine the possibility of a CAPD in children. For the past nine years, researchers have also been applying knowledge of CANS function to the optimal fitting of hearing aids (Del Polito, Smith & Dempsey, 1980; Franklin, 1975; 1980; 1981; Hayes & Jerger, 1979; McSpaden, 1982; Shirinian & Arnst, 1982; Young & Protti, 1981). The fitting of a hearing aid entails an in-depth analysis of the individual's communication potential. Therefore, one's ability to hear sound as well as to interpret the speech message is of utmost importance. Since sound will be directed through a mechanical device that is not as distortion free as the *normal* ear, the quality of the sound source and knowledge of the status of the CANS is important. If one aids an individual whose central auditory pathways are deficient, that individual will most likely not be as successful a candidate for hearing-aid use as the individual with an intact CANS.

Some audiologists disagree with this concept, however, and do not feel that evaluation of the CANS for optimal hearing aid fitting has sufficient value (LaMarche & Rudmin, 1982). Nevertheless, the vast majority of researchers who have reported on this subject have concurred with the justification of evaluating the CANS prior to a hearing aid evaluation and subsequent hearing aid fitting.

Several approaches have been advocated for assessing CANS status for the purpose of hearing aid evaluation. Franklin (1975; 1980; 1981) uses a filtered version of Fairbanks Rhyme Test in which the high-frequency energies and the low-frequency energies of the stimuli are presented to opposite ears. Her procedure was based on her observation that hearing-impaired individuals were able to discriminate consonants when low-band pass information and high-band pass information was presented to opposite ears. She found that scores were reduced when both low-band and high-band information was presented to the same ear.

Franklin suggests that the right ear should receive the high-frequency emphasis hearing aid and the left ear should be fit with an extended low-frequency emphasis instrument. The reason for this is based on the belief that the left hemisphere (right ear) is dominant for consonant identification whereas the right hemisphere (left ear) is dominant for prosodic features of speech that include rhythm, intonation and pitch.

Weber (1977) also encourages split-band fitting of hearing aids for hearing-impaired individuals. He recommends that patients with binaural sensorineural hearing loss wear high-frequency amplification on the right ear and a low-frequency emphasis instrument on the left ear for optimal speech discrimination. Weber's recommendation is similar to Franklin's in advising that dichotic fitting of hearing aids be implemented for bilateral hearing impairments. However, he does not indicate whether or not he evaluates the status of the CANS prior to the hearing-aid fitting.

Young and Protti (1981) also advocate dichotic fitting of hearing aids in children. However, they feel that prior assessment of the status of the CANS is necessary, reasoning that such assessment provides the knowledge for determining the desirability of monaural or binaural amplification. Tests of central auditory function, which they used to provide the basis for such decisions, were the Competing Sentence Test and the Filtered Speech Test from the Willeford Central Auditory Test Battery and Katz' SSW Test. They utilize the test results to determine which ear should be fit if aided monaurally and, if the child is to be fit binaurally, which ear should receive the low-frequency information and which ear the high-frequency information. Young and Protti believe that the ear that is dominant on the above mentioned tests should receive amplification in monaural fittings. If a dichotic fitting seems to be appropriate, the dominant ear, as measured by central auditory tests, should receive the high-pass band or high-frequency emphasis aid and the opposite ear should receive the low-pass band or extended low-frequency instrument.

Shirinian and Arnst (1982) have also suggested that the status of the central auditory pathway is important in determining which ear or ears to fit with amplification. They report that central auditory function decreases with age and that hearing aid performance was better in the ear with the best CAP test performance. They also noted that the right ear showed a greater magnitude of central aging effect. This fact argues for CAP tests during hearing-aid evaluations to allow for more judiciously applied monaural and dichotic fittings. Hayes and Jerger (1979) concur.

Since 1977, the authors have been evaluating the status of the CANS prior to a hearing aid evaluation in an effort to determine which amplification arrangement would be most appropriate for a hearing-impaired individual. We have been using Sinha's (1959) technique of presenting speech in white noise ipsilaterally under earphones at 40 dB SL re the PTA and at a signal-to-noise ratio of either 0 dB or +6 dB. Routinely, we have used either the W-22 word discrimination lists or NU-6 discrimination lists for individuals with mental ages of eight years or greater. For younger children, discrimination lists are selected that are appropriate for the mental and/or language age of the child. It has been our observation that information regarding the status of the CANS can even be obtained while using an informal discrimination list for very young children with limited vocabulary. We utilize the speech-in-white-noise technique when an individual demonstrates a bilaterally symmetrical, sensorineural hearing loss. Our primary objective is to assess the difference in scores obtained for right and left ears.

This technique is very expeditious and generally yields good information for the selection of monaural or binaural amplification. In instances where the speech-in-white-noise technique does not adequately demonstrate ear differences, additional CAP tests are employed.

The results we have obtained with the speech-in-white-noise paradigm have been quite favorable; examples are shown in Table 39. We observed that ear differences obtained under earphones for speech-in-

Table 39
Speech scores for aided and unaided listening in quiet and white noise conditions

Subject	Ear	Unaided in Quiet	Unaided in Noise	Aided in Quiet	Aided in Noise
RW	RE	82	52	84	76
	LE	84	78	84	84
GM	RE	82	70	100	84
	LE	86	64	100	68
LC	RE	88	56	90	50
	LE	92	68	92	72
SJ	RE	94	58	92	72
	LE	90	72	90	92
JS	RE	80	36	80	72
	LE	88	44	80	84

Signal-to-noise ratio = 0 dB

white-noise were less dramatic when compared to the individuals' aided performance in noise in the sound field. A difference between ears for speech-in-white-noise of only eight percent often produced marked differences between aided performance when amplification was alternated between ears in a complex listening environment (S/N = 0). Also, our clients invariably noticed a difference in the quality of sound between the two ears, with the quality being better in the ear with the least amount of central involvement or better speech-in-white-noise results.

For the past seven years we have realized the importance of assessing the central nervous system prior to a hearing-aid evaluation. Now with the rapid growth of the in-the-ear hearing aid industry, the ability to select which ear processes auditory information in noise most efficiently is of increasing importance. The time it takes to assess this function is well worth the effort, for such an assessment can help the audiologist in selecting an optimal hearing aid arrangement.

8

Case Studies

The following case study summaries are presented to illustrate further the wide variety of children with central auditory problems that were implied by the data presented in Chapter 1. In each instance, results would not have been predicted without central auditory assessments. Consequently, management protocols and attitudes toward the children and their families were modified in significantly favorable ways.

CASE ONE—DELAYED IDENTIFICATION OF A
CENTRAL AUDITORY PROCESSING DISORDER

DS, a nine-year-old, was initially seen for speech and hearing evaluation at the age of two years. The major complaint was a w-r substitution, which was confirmed. He was also found to have a slight fluency problem and a mild expressive-language dysfunction. Except for a 35 dB impairment at 8000 Hz in each ear, his hearing was found to be normal, although he had numerous episodes of otitis media between the ages of one and two years, and PE tubes were inserted on three different occasions. Three years of speech and language therapy followed in two different states, after which he was reevaluated. This evaluation resulted in a similar diagnosis to the one made three years earlier. At this time, he still had the w-r substitution and a slight fluency problem. Auditory perception "was not formally assessed, but appeared normal to the examining clinician." Numerous other tests revealed normal language performance and a normal IQ. DS had also had two neurological examinations between his first and second speech and language evaluations, both of which resulted in normal findings.

Four years later, DS was referred to our clinic for a CAP evaluation. Although he had received two more years of therapy for "expressive" problems, the major complaint was that he was now having academic difficulties at school. Specifically, he was falling behind expected levels in mathematics, science, and social studies, despite being a good reader. His case history revealed that he was easily frustrated, had a short attention span, lacked confidence and motivation, was easily confused, and had problems following directions. His teacher stated that he was a slow starter, that he failed to complete assignments, and that she considered him an underachiever.

In discourse with DS, it was apparent that he had difficulty comprehending conversation, and his CAP test results revealed the probable reason. He was given 11 CAP tests and failed all of them. He scored below the normal range for nine-year-olds on all four of the tests in the Willeford Battery. He showed a similar performance on all three tasks of the IC-CS of male vs. female voices, the Compressed WIPI, the SSI-ICM, the Pitch-Pattern Sequence Test, and Masking Level Differences.

On the basis of this knowledge, and with counseling of the parents and school personnel, DS was assigned to a self-contained classroom and a "patient and understanding" teacher, both of which helped immediately. His academic problems have decreased, except in discussion-type classes, where group interactions continue to confuse him.

CASE TWO—SPEECH, LANGUAGE, AND CENTRAL AUDITORY PROCESSING ASSESSMENT

DR, a ten-year-old fourth-grader, was referred because of social problems and school performance described by his adoptive (at age five and a half months) mother as a "disaster." Of further concern was the parent's belief that he had begun to speak more softly and less distinctly during the past two years. He began walking, or rather running, according to his mother, at seven months. He never went through a crawling stage. He began saying words like "dada," "cookie," "water," and "go" at 9 months and was toilet trained at 15 months. At the time of evaluation, DR was in an *open* classroom, in which he was doing poorly in mathematics and science and seldom finished his assignments. His teacher described him as immature, very distractible, and a serious discipline problem in the classroom. Nevertheless, he was functioning above age-level for language. His syntactic and semantic sentence competence was rated as good, and he had no fluency, articulation, or phonatory problems. A "quick learner," he began to read at 3½ years of age and was characterized as a good reader. He displayed rare musical talent, playing classical music on the piano by the age of four.

At the age of three years, DR was seen by a psychiatrist who diagnosed brain damage on the basis of grossly abnormal EEG patterns. Diffuse and spike/wave activity were observed, with polyspike discharges arising bisynchronously over both hemispheres, but somewhat more from the frontal cortex. He was placed on ritalin. He was later evaluated by a pediatrician who noted seizures and changed the medication to dilantin. Subsequently, upon being examined by a neuropsychologist, it was noted that DR was being given dexedrine.

Referral was ultimately made by the neuropsychologist who described DR as a bright-normal youngster who was hyperactive, restless, could not sleep, commonly experienced nightmares, had social problems, had a poor self-image, and had no close friends. At one point he was dismissed from a nursery school because he was a disruptive influence. The neuropsychologist referred DR for a

CAP evaluation because he appeared to have inordinate difficulty comprehending her speech—English with a Swiss accent. Although he had a history of difficulty in understanding complex speech, or listening in "active" environments and groups, he usually did well in one-to-one conversations.

Prior to the CAP assessment DR was given a speech and language evaluation. Results revealed a Peabody IQ score of 108 and speech and language skills generally at or above his chronological age. His memory for sentences, Lindamood Auditory Conceptualization performance, and ITPA Auditory Subtest scores were all at age level or above. These results were in agreement with those administered at school.

DR was then seen for the CAP evaluation. The results on the Willeford Battery revealed severely abnormal BF performance at both 30 dB and 40 dB SL. Other behavioral CAP test scores were within normal limits. He was reevaluated three months later with essentially identical results. At that time his mother reported that our recommended management strategies had resulted in encouraging relationships at home and in his academic performance at school. She noted that individualized assistance in mathematics had brought dramatic improvement in that subject.

CASE THREE—HEREDITY IN CENTRAL AUDITORY PROCESSING DISORDERS

CW, a six-year-old second-grader, was referred because of problems similar to those experienced by the mother and maternal grandmother. Those problems included difficulty in school, where poor reading skills caused the mother to struggle academically, even though she maintained that she liked to read and had a reasonably good attitude about school. She had required a great deal of tutoring, except in mathematics, which was her favorite subject. CW was a breech-born, premature baby who had breathing complications. She developed normally until 18 months of age, then began to drop slowly behind for reasons unknown, and she frequently had colic during that period. Between the ages of three and six years, she fainted several times for undetermined causes. Exceptional behaviors at school included social isolation, distractability, poor concentration, short attention span, poor eye-hand coordination, and fatigue. Both the mother and grandmother identified with these problems, which they felt were similar to their own experiences, both as children and in their subsequent adult lives as well.

CW's CAP performance on the Willeford Battery showed large asymmetries on the CS, FS, and BF Tests (the latter at each of several SLs), and on the Compressed WIPI Test (Beasley et al, 1976). Both the 31-year-old mother and the 58-year-old grandmother were later tested at their request and both scored abnormally on the same tests as CW, except for the CS test, on which both scored normally.

These findings lend support to hereditary factors as a cause for CAP. CW was reevaluated 13 months later with the identical pattern of results and, although she showed a slight improvement on the CS test, a result suggesting that maturation had occurred for that function, the great difference between the scores for her two ears remained. Nonetheless, her mother reported that CW was showing gratifying response to the compensatory management program that was outlined for them.

CASE FOUR—OTITIS MEDIA OR CENTRAL AUDITORY PROCESSING DISORDER?

RN is a nine-year-old boy who has had repeated bouts of otitis media since infancy and still has them. He repeated first grade and has always had trouble learning at school. He is restless, distractable, and inattentive, for which he has taken various medications (ritalin, etc.). He has particular difficulty with reading, seemingly a family trait on the mother's side, since she and two of her brothers are poor readers and demonstrated the other behaviors that characterize RN when they were in school.

This boy was receiving special reading assistance at school and showing no progress. Upon hearing that we were experimenting with ear-occlusion techniques to seek improvement in auditory figure-ground listening, school personnel had the boy wear protective earmuffs during special instruction periods. No referral for diagnosis of CAP problems had been made. However, he continued to experience classroom difficulty.

Upon eventual referral for CAP evaluation, RN was found to have a mild, flat, conductive hearing loss and Type B tympanograms in both ears, suggesting the presence of middle-ear fluid. The conductive hearing impairment, coupled with the wearing of sound-occluding ear-muffs, combined with poor reading skills, appeared to be the causes of many of the boy's behaviors and learning problems at school. We referred him to an otologist. Nonetheless, before doing so we did perform a series of CAP tests on him. He scored within normal limits on the four tests in the Willeford Battery and also on the Compressed WIPI Test. Two messages seem clear from this case: (1) obtain a proper diagnosis before applying behavior-altering treatment, and (2) CAPD does not appear to be an inevitable result of early and prolonged otitis media.

CASE FIVE—A GIFTED CHILD WITH A CENTRAL AUDITORY PROCESSING DISORDER

MP, an 8-year-old female with an IQ at the 99th percentile, was seen for a CAP evaluation due to her parents' concern regarding her auditory behavior. MP is a precocious child who comes from a very intellectually-endowed family. Her 12-year-old brother is a university freshman in computer science. MP began reading and writing and could perform addition, subtraction, and integer computations before her third birthday. By 4½, she was reading for pleasure and could perform all four arithmetic operations with ease. Because MP was 12 days too young for kindergarten in a rigidly oriented, age-graded school, placement was delayed until age 5 ½. MP attended her kindergarten class one day before she decided to leave the classroom by herself, in the middle of class, and walk through a driving rain to her home two miles away. She absolutely refused to go back to school that year. A year later, although excited about attending first grade, MP became quickly discouraged and said she was not learning anything. A very understanding principal allowed her to attend classes from first to sixth grade depending upon her particular performance level in various subject areas. Throughout this time, teachers and her parents were concerned with her "inattentiveness." She had particular problems understanding English spoken with a British accent, even though she had lived in Canada and was frequently exposed to that accent.

MP's CAP performance showed decreased ability with both cortical and subcortical function tests. Poor performance was noted on the Compressed WIPI Test, the CS and BF Tests from the Willeford Battery. MP was tested two years later, with similar results on all tests, except for an improvement in performance for the left ear on the CS Test. This improvement in scores is often seen for the left ear with a dichotic test and is probably due to the maturation of the CANS.

Reports from MP's mother indicate that MP is coping well with her problem. Mrs. P writes that "knowing MP has an auditory processing problem is the biggest part of her own coping. . . ." MP is using compensatory techniques in aiding her listening skills in her everyday environment.

CASE SIX—JUVENILE DELINQUENCY AND CENTRAL AUDITORY PROCESSING DISORDERS

BR is an 18-year-old male who has encountered serious difficulties with the law. At the time of the CAP evaluation, he was serving a probation sentence for homicide. A court order directed him to a psychiatrist, who then sent him to our clinic for CAP evaluation. BR had academic difficulties throughout school. Upon finishing high school, he had hopes of enlisting in the Army. This goal was denied, however, when he was rejected for military service. So, he proceeded to form his "own army." He directed combat drills and, on one of these maneuvers, accidentally shot a companion.

BR's CAP results showed decreased performance on a sub-cortical level test. He scored far below the normal range of function on the BF Test of the Willeford Battery. His performance on cortical level tests was within the normal range of function.

Throughout BR's life, he has had difficulty with impulsive behavior, attention problems, and distractability. Although it is difficult to determine to what extent, it appears that a CAPD may have been a significant contributor to the problems in BR's life.

CASE SEVEN—MANAGEMENT STRATEGIES IN
CENTRAL AUDITORY PROCESSING DISORDERS

Rk, a seven-year-old male, was seen for CAP evaluation because of his failure to progress adequately in his academic setting. As reported by his third grade teacher, RK was highly distractible and had difficulty succeeding at practically any academic task. Completing assignments was a rarity for RK, and he often sat rolling a pencil on his desk after instructions were given. He acted as if he did not understand even the simplest of classroom instructions.

Upon referral for a CAP evaluation, RK was found to have a CAPD, scoring below the normal range on Willeford's CS and FS Tests. Following the evaluation, specific recommendations were suggested in an effort to aid RK in his academic classroom setting. During desk activities, earmuffs were suggested in an attempt to attenuate classroom noise. Also, during classroom instruction, RK utilized a mild gain FM auditory trainer. Not only did his performance on academic work improve, but RK also demonstrated definite improvements in his overall work behavior. His attention skills improved along with his ability to complete assignments.

Appendix

Tape-Recorded Tests: Care and Use

All of the audiological tests discussed in this chapter, and some of those discussed under speech-language measures, are recorded on magnetic tape. The primary purpose of recording a test on tape is to provide greater consistency of the test stimuli when they are presented to different patients or patient populations than can be achieved with variable live-voice presentations. It is important that, even when taped signals are employed, other variables such as stimulus-presentation levels, instrumentation, and test environment be held constant (Willeford & Billger, 1978). Even when test stimuli are recorded on tape and played back on proper tape decks in controlled environments with standardized presentation protocols, there are still important pitfalls to avoid. These problems are discussed in the following pages.

DUPLICATING FROM A MASTER TAPE

Regardless of the nature of the stimuli on the Master (original) Tape, the duplications generated from it should be accurate representations of the acoustic characteristics of the Master. Of course, that means the studio or business firm that undertakes the production of duplicate tapes should use good quality tape and record-playback instrumentation and observe a standard protocol in the duplication procedure. The lack of such quality control and standardization can reduce the consistency among duplications and jeopardize accurate comparisons of test results obtained from the duplicate to normative data produced from the Master Tape. The consistency of a duplicated tape can be reasonably assessed by the tedious procedure of monitoring the VU-meter peaks of the tape's calibration tone and subsequent test stimuli. Differences between stimuli, or between tapes, can be reliably identified in this manner. That, of course, is a fundamental purpose of a peak-reading VU meter. Recording the values of signal peaks can also serve as a means for monitoring deteriorating signals on a given tape over time. This should be done routinely with clinical and research tapes so that one can be aware of changes in the taped signals. When changes in the signals are noted, that tape should either be replaced or else the test's norms should be reestablished for that particular tape.

It is possible, of course, to assess the electroacoustic characteristics of taped signals, but that is time consuming and, if one contracts for such services, expensive. Real-time electronic analyses can be performed on all or selected segments of a series of recordings to compare their acoustic features. The authors recently employed this approach by arrangement with the Trane Engineering, Mechanics, and Acoustics Laboratory of La Crosse, Wisconsin. They analyzed the sound level consistency of a series of new and used (some as old as three years) sequentially duplicated tapes. Analyses were performed for the calibration tone and for several stimulus points in each channel of the dual channel tapes. Using a digitalizing rate of 20,000 samples/second for each channel, they determined that there was excellent consistency among the sample tapes. The maximum sound-pressure-level (SPL) difference among the new tapes was only 0.53 dB and, except for a 4.39 dB difference at one data point, the greatest difference between any of the data points on the older (used) tapes and the mean of the new tapes was 2.79 dB. The detailed SPL data are shown in Tables 40 and 41.

We have found it surprising that most people we have contacted in the tape and recording industry neither rely on, have access to, nor believe in the necessity for such means of monitoring the fidelity of recordings. The same seems to be true for university Electrical Engineering and Audio-Visual Departments. Of course, duplications under any

Table 40
Maximum SPL differences among 1984 tapes*

Data Points		1984 Tapes			Maximum dB Difference
		1	2	3	
1	(THERE)—	6.71	6.53	6.55	.15
2	(WAS)—	5.18	5.28	5.18	.10
3	(FROST)—	6.43	6.53	6.28	.25[†]
4	(ON)—	5.82	5.93	5.82	.11
5	(THE)—	6.13	6.08	6.13	.05
6	(GROUND)—	6.13	5.93	6.13	.20

*Duplicated simultaneously on slave recording units from Master Tape.
†Maximum data-point difference between tapes.

Table 41

SPL values re. calibration tone for six data points on six
different tapes. Values represent real-time analysis run
at a digitalizing rate of 20,000 samples/second

Data Points		Tape					
		1 (1984)	2 (1984)	3 (1984)	4 (5/82)	5 (8/82)	6 (10/80)
1	(THERE)—	6.71	6.53	6.55	7.99	6.12	8.16
2	(WAS)—	5.18	5.28	5.18	6.17	4.68	6.79
3	(FROST)—	6.43	6.53	6.28	8.44	5.75	7.50
4	(ON)—	5.82	5.93	5.82	7.51	4.24	6.61
5	(THE)—	6.13	6.08	6.13	7.99	5.10	7.33
6	(GROUND)—	6.13	5.93	6.13	8.22	5.36	7.33

circumstances should be done on good quality, low-noise tape on which
the polyester or acetate base is coated with tiny bits of magnetic material,
usually iron oxide or chromium dioxide. While some variability in the
evenness of these magnetic particles may occur, their distribution on
good quality tapes is relatively similar. Small differences in intensity
levels are of little consequence for most taped tests since they are normally played at fairly high sensation levels. Discussions of the technical
aspects of tape recording may be found in Manly (1979), Jorgensen (1980),
and Carver (1983). Occasionally, good information is available in the
owner's manual supplied with tape recorders. Encyclopedias also offer
fundamental and detailed treatments of the principles of tape recording.
One of the most popular sources for knowledge about tape recording and
recorders may be found in *Tape Guide*, a regular feature of the magazine,
Audio, in which readers' questions about tape-related problems are
answered by one of the magazine's contributing editors.*

CARE AND MAINTENANCE OF TAPE RECORDERS

Although problems may occur to cause inconsistencies in duplications of magnetic tape recordings, such difficulties should be minimized
when duplications are run with the same instrumentation from the same
master copy. It is more likely that alterations occur in tape recordings that
are the result of poor maintenance of the tape itself and that of the tape
recorder used as the playback instrument. The pitfalls to be avoided may
be found in the sources cited above and in Roberson (1982). The latter is
highly recommended. Some of the major problems follow.

Audio, 1515 Broadway, New York, N.Y. 10036.

Magnetized Tapedeck Components

Tape heads and other metal objects in the tape path (e.g., guides, capstans, and tension arms) incur magnetic buildup over time. This may result from continued passage of the tape laden with its tiny magnetic particles, from transient magnetisms resulting from starting and stopping the unit, or from exposure to other magnetic fields such as shortwave radios, television sets, speakers, and transformers. Tapes exposed to a magnetized tapedeck or to other magnetic fields are vulnerable to erasure of their magnetic signals, particularly the high frequencies that do not penetrate the tape as deeply as do the middle and low frequencies (Burstein, 1982). The subjective effect is that the recording will begin to sound dull. Carver (1983) observes that increasing tape "hiss" noise is a result of magnetized heads and contributes further to degradation of taped signals. The solution to such dangers is to avoid exposing recorded tapes to extraneous magnetic fields and to periodically demagnetize one's tapedeck. The instruments and proper procedures for this process may be found in the above references, or with instructions available with demagnetizing devices.

Cleanliness

Both the magnetic surface of recorded tapes and the tapedeck should be kept clean. Fingers contain oils, soil, and perspiration, which can cause alterations in the quality of the signal through dropout and fluttering. Thus, one should avoid touching the magnetic surface of tapes. It is also important that playback heads, capstans, and pinch rollers be cleaned after every four or five playings using cleaning liquid for reel tapes or cassette cleaners for cassettes. Cleaning supplies are available at commercial establishments. Dirt and dust that collect on the parts of the recorder over time can diminish the quality of tape-recorded tests, especially those that involve sensitive or degraded stimuli such as filtered speech, dichotic CVs, binaural fusion, and compressed speech. Signal dropout and buildup of tape noise also result from unclean recorder parts that dilute the quality of recorded materials. When not in use, tapes should be carefully rewound (to avoid creasing) and stored in the box, a plastic bag, or wherever they will be free of dust and dirt. Tapes should also be stored in a location that will prevent their exposure to high or low temperatures, excessive humidity, and direct sunlight.

All of the above recommendations should be followed in order to avoid deterioration of the tape and, consequently, in the quality of the recorded material. Even with good care, however, tapes that are used frequently lose their quality over time and should be replaced if they are expected to conform to the test's norms as suggested earlier. Thus, possible changes in the quality of tapes should be monitored regularly.

The use of second or third generation tapes (copies) has become a common practice, but it should be avoided in all instances where the tapes are to be used for clinical or research purposes. Taped clinical tests should be duplicated from a high-quality master tape only. Each tape generation further dilutes the quality of its content material. One should also be aware that duplication of some taped materials may be a violation of copyright laws. Even with uncopyrighted materials, ethically, one should gain permission from the author prior to duplication.

Head Alignment

When playback recorder heads are misaligned, it means that only part of the recorded signal is transduced. Consequently, there will be reduction in the signal amplitude (level). Moreover, in stereo tapes, the two tracks containing the stereo signals may be out of alignment with each other. This causes a time difference between playback-signal channels (Carver, 1983; Jorgensen, 1980; Manly, 1979; Roberson, 1982).

General Tape-Use Protocol

There are a number of factors about playing recorded tapes that, experience has shown, do not seem to be common knowledge. One factor is tape-tapedeck compatibility that has to do with tape-track width among reel-type tapes. For example, playing a two-track (half-track) recording on a four-track (quarter-track) playback deck results in the narrower four-track heads "reading" only part of the wider two-track magnetic signals. A partial loss of signal is inevitable from that mismatch, with a consequent diminution of the signal's fidelity. Signal deterioration is minimal when a four-track tape is played on a two-track recorder. Better recording quality is obtained with two-track tapes but, unfortunately, the great majority of reel-type recorders utilized in most clinical settings in recent years are four-track units. However, the current trend in the tape industry is toward the use of cassettes (estimated to be about 70 percent among audiologists performing CAP tests), so that tape-tapedeck compatibility concerns are circumvented. Other general tape use factors include: (1) the necessity for properly calibrating the tape circuits; (2) setting test calibration tones with the assistance of VU-meter readings, after which channel gain-levels should not be altered to compensate for frequency-filtering or other modifications in the test's signals; and (3) compensation for the drop in signal intensities when stereo tapes are played through audiometers that do not have two full channels. In that instance, its signals are split and a reduction in energy occurs in each product.

All of the foregoing factors must be observed if the advantages of tape-recorded tests are to remain.

REFERENCES

Aaron P (1981). Diagnosis and remediation of learning disabilities in children—a neuropsychological key approach. In Hynd G & Obrzut J (Eds.), *Neuropsychological assessment and the school-age child.* New York: Grune & Stratton, 303–333

Allen D, Bliss L, & Timmons J (1981). Language evaluation: science or art? *Journal of Speech and Hearing Disorders, 46,* 66–68

Aman M (1980). Psychotropic drugs and learning problems—a selective review. *Journal of Learning Disabilities, 13(12),* 36–46

American Speech, Language, and Hearing Association (1982). Joint committee on infant hearing statement. *ASHA, 24,* 1017–1018

Arnst D, & Katz J (1982). *Central auditory assessment: the SSW test.* San Diego: College-Hill Press

Aten J (1972). Auditory memory and auditory sequencing. *Proceedings of the First Annual Memphis State University Symposium on Auditory Processing and Learning Disabilities, 135,* 108–135

Ayres A (1972). *Sensory integration and learning disorders.* Los Angeles: Western Psychological Services

Baker H, & Leland B (1935, 1967 [Rev.]) *Detroit tests of learning aptitude.* Indianapolis: Bobbs-Merrill

Barnes W, Magoun H, & Ranson S (1943) Ascending auditory pathway in the brainstem of monkey. *Journal of Comparative Neurology, 79,* 129–152

Barr D (1972). *Auditory perceptual disorders.* Springfield, IL: Charles C. Thomas

Baru A, & Karaseva T (1972). *The brain and hearing.* New York: Consultants Bureau

Beasley D, & Freeman B (1977). Time-altered speech as a measure of central auditory processing. In Keith R (Ed.), *Central auditory dysfunction.* New York; Grune & Stratton, 129–173

Beasley D, Maki J, & Orchik D (1976). Children's perception of time-compressed speech using two measures of speech discrimination. *Journal of Speech and Hearing Disorders, 41,* 216–225

Beasley D, & Rintelmann A (1979) Central auditory processing. In Rintelmann W (Ed.), *Hearing assessment.* Baltimore: University Park Press, 321–349

Behrmann P (undated). *Activities for developing auditory perception.* San Rafael, CA: Academic Therapy Publications

Bekesy G (1960). *Experiments in hearing.* New York: McGraw-Hill

Bell J (1980). Ritalin and children: miracle drug or menace? *Family Weekly Magazine*. Fort Collins: Colorado. November 2

Berlin C, Hughes L, Lowe-Bell S, & Berlin H (1973). Dichotic right ear advantage in children 5 to 13. *Cortex, 9*, 394–402

Berlin C, & Lowe S (1972). Temporal and dichotic factors in central auditory testing. In Katz J (Ed.), *Handbook of clinical audiology* (ed 1). Baltimore: Williams & Wilkins, 280–312

Berlin C, & McNeil M (1976). Dichotic listening. In Lass N (Ed.), *Contemporary issues in experimental phonetics*. New York: Academic Press, 327–388

Berman A (1976). The link between learning-disabilities and juvenile delinquency. Office of Juvenile Delinquency and Delinquency Prevention, Law Enforcement Assistance Administration, Washington, D.C., April

Berman A, & Siegal A (1976). Adaptive and learning skills in juvenile delinquents: a neuropsychological analysis. *Journal of Learning Disabilities, 9*, 583–595

Block N (1983). Mental pictures and cognitive science. *Philosophical Review, 92*, 499–541

Bocca E, Calearo C, & Cassinari V (1954). A new method for testing hearing in temporal lobe tumors. *Acta Otolaryngolica, 44*, 219–221

Bocca E, & Calearo C (1963). Central hearing processes. In Jerger J (Ed.), *Modern developments in audiology* (ed 1). New York: Academic Press, 337–370

Brodal A, (1969). *Neurological anatomy–in relation to clinical medicine* (ed. 2). Oxford: Oxford University Press

Broman S, (1983). Obstetric medications. In C Brown (Ed.), *Childhood learning disabilities and prenatal risk*. New Jersey: Johnson and Johnson Baby Products Company Pediatric Round Table, 9, 56–64

Brugge J (1975). Progress in neuroanatomy and neurophysiology of auditory cortex. In Eagles E (Ed.), *The nervous system*, Vol. 3. *Human communication and its disorders*. New York: Raven Press, 97–111

Brunt M (1978). The staggered spondaic word test. In Katz J (Ed.), *Handbook of clinical audiology* (ed 2). Baltimore: Williams & Wilkins, 262–275

Burleigh A, Skinner B, & Norris T (1982). Central auditory processing disorders in children: a five-year study. Paper presented at the American Speech, Language, and Hearing Association Convention, Toronto, Ontario

Burns G, & Watson, B (1973). Factor analysis of the revised I.T.P.A. with underachieving children. *Journal of Learning Disabilities, 6*, 371–376

Burstein H (1982). Tape guide. *Audio, 66(8)*, 24

Butler K (1975). Short-course on auditory perception. Presented at the American Speech and Hearing Association Convention, Washington, D.C.

Butler K (1980). Disorders of other aspects of auditory function. In VanHattum R (Ed.), *Communication disorders*. New York: MacMillan Publishing, 123–158

Butler K, Hedrick D, & Manning C (1973). *Composite auditory perceptual test.* Hayward, CA: Alameda County School Department

Carhart R (1967). Audiologic tests: questions and speculations. In McConnell F, Ward P (Eds.), *Deafness in childhood*. Nashville: Vanderbilt University Press, 229–251

Carpenter M (1972). *Core text of neuroanatomy*. Baltimore: Williams & Wilkins

Carver W (1983). Tape recording and tape recorders: Their care and maintenance. *Seminars in Hearing, 4,* 311–315

Chandler H, & Jones K (1983). Learning disabled or emotionally disturbed: Does it make any difference? Part 1. *Journal of Learning Disabilities, 16,* 432–434

Chow K (1951). Numerical estimates of the auditory central nervous system of the rhesus monkey. *Journal of Comparative Neurology, 95,* 159–175

Cole R (1977). Invariant features and feature detectors: some developmental implications. In Segalowitz S & Gruber F (Eds.), *Language development and neurological theory.* New York: Academic Press, 319–345

Costello M (1977). Evaluation of auditory behavior of children using the Flowers-Costello test of central auditory abilities. In Keith R (Ed.), *Central auditory dysfunction.* New York: Grune & Stratton, 257–276

Craig D (1979). Neuropsychological assessment in public psychiatric hospitals: the current state of practice. *Clinical Neuropsychology, 1,* 1–7

Crosby E, Humphrey T, & Lauer E (1962). *Correlative anatomy of the nervous system.* New York: MacMillan

Curtiss S (1977). *Genie: a psycholinguistic study of a modern-day "wild-child."* New York: Academic Press, 1977

Del Polito G, Smith D, & Dempsey C (1980). Central auditory testing: implications for hearing aid candidacy. In Libby E (Ed.), *Binaural hearing and amplification,* Vol. 1. Chicago: Zenetron, 201–216

De Renzi E, & Vignola L (1962). The token test: a sensitive test to detect receptive disturbances in aphasics. *Brain, 85,* 665–678

Dimond S (1976). Drugs to improve learning in man: implications and neuro-psychological analysis. In R Knights & D Bakker (Eds.), *The neuropsychology of learning disorders.* Baltimore: University Park Press, 367–379

Dobie R, & Berlin C (1979). Influence of otitis media on hearing and development. In otitis media and child development: Speech, language and education. *Annals of Otology, Rhinology, & Laryngology,* supplement 60, part 2, *88 (5),* 48–53

Downs D, & Crum M (1978). Processing demands during auditory learning under degraded listening conditions. *Journal of Speech and Hearing Research, 21,* 702–714

Duchan J, & Katz J (1983). Language and auditory processing: top down plus bottom up. In E Lasky & J Katz (Eds.), *Central auditory processing disorders.* Baltimore: University Park Press, 31–45

Duffy F, Burchfiel J, & Lambroso C (1980). Brain electrical activity mapping (BEAM): a new method for extending the clinical utility of EEG and evoked potential data. *Annals of Neurology, 5,* 309–321

Dzick D (1967). Vision and the juvenile delinquent. *Journal of American Optometric Association, 37(5),* A Symposium on Juvenile Delinquency, B'Nai B-rith, Stanley Lachman, Lodge #446, 2nd annual Symposium on Juvenile Delinquency, Chattanooga, Tenn. April 6. (Available from American Optometric Association Library).

Eden K, Green J, & Hansen J (1973). *Auditory training.* Iowa City: University of Iowa Campus Stores

Ehrlich C (1978). A case history for children. In J Katz (Ed.), *Handbook of clinical audiology* (ed 2). Baltimore: Williams & Wilkins, 388–396

Erulkar S (1959). The responses of single units of the inferior colliculus of the cat to acoustic stimulation. *Proceedings of the Royal Society: London*, Series B, *150*, 336–355

Ferry P, Culbertson J, Fitzgibbons P, & Netsky M (1979). Hemispheric asymmetry and specialization. *International Journal of Pediatric Otorhinolaryngology, 1*, 13–24

Fisher L (1976). Fisher's auditory problems checklist. Bemidji, Minnesota: Life Products

Flowers A, Costello M, & Small V (1970) *Manual for Flowers-Costello test of central auditory abilities*. Dearborn, Michigan: Perceptual Learning Systems

Forbes A & Morison B (1938). Cortical responses to sensory stimulation under deep barbituate narcosis. *Journal of Neurophysiology, 2*, 112–128

Franklin B (1975). The effect of combining low and high-frequency passbands on consonant recognition in the hearing-impaired. *Journal of Speech and Hearing Research, 18*, 719–727

Franklin B (1980). Split band amplification. In E Libby (Ed.), *Binaural hearing aid amplification*, Vol. 2. Chicago: Zenetron, 311–322

Franklin B (1981). Split-band amplification: a hi/lo hearing aid fitting. *Ear and Hearing, 2*, 230–233

Freeman B, & Beasley D (1976). *Performance of reading-impaired and normal reading children on time-compressed monosyllabic and sentential stimuli*, paper presented at the American Speech and Hearing Association Convention, Houston

French J (1957). The reticular formation. *Scientific American, 196*, 54–60

Gaddes W (1978). Learning disabilities: the search for causes. Learning Disabilities: Information Please, *Canadian Association of Learning Disabilities*, 1–8

Gadow K (1983). Effects of stimulant drugs on academic performance in hyperactive and learning disabled children. *Journal of Learning Disabilities, 16(5)*, 290–299

Galambos R (1956). Some recent experiments on the neurophysiology of hearing. *Annals of Otology, Rhinology, and Laryngology, 65*, 1055

Gallagher A, Tobey E, Cullen J, & Rampp D (1976). An investigation of c-v and digit recall with children failing auditory processing portions of a speech and language screening test, paper presented at the American Speech and Hearing Association Convention, Houston

Gazzaniga M, & LeDoux J (1978). *The integrated mind*. New York: Plenum Press

Gearheart B (1977). *Learning disabilities—educational strategies* (ed 2). St. Louis: C. V. Mosby

Gearheart B (1981). *Learning disabilities—educational strategies* (ed 3). St. Louis: C. V. Mosby

Geschwind N (1968). Neurological foundations of language. In H Myklebust (Ed.), *Progress in learning disabilities*, Vol. 1. New York: Grune & Stratton, 182–198

Geschwind N (1979). Specializations of the human brain. *Scientific American, 241*, 180–199

Geschwind N, & Behan P (1982). Left-handedness: association with immune disease, migraine, and developmental learning disorders. *Proceedings of the National Academy of Science, 79,* 5097–5100

Gesell A, & Amatruda C (1947). *Developmental diagnosis.* New York: Paul B. Hoeber

Gillet P (1974). *Auditory processes.* San Rafael, CA: Academic Therapy Publications

Glasier J (1981). An analysis of central auditory function in emotionally disturbed children. Unpublished paper

Glattke T (1978). Anatomy and physiology of the auditory system (ed 2). In D Rose (Ed.), *Audiological assessment.* Englewood Cliffs, NJ: Prentice-Hall, 22–51

Goldberg J, & Moore R (1967). Ascending projections of the lateral lemniscus in the cat and monkey. *Journal of Comparative Neurology, 129,* 143–156

Goldman R, Fristoe M, & Woodcock R (1970). *Test of auditory discrimination.* Circle Pines, Minnesota: American Guidance Service

Goldman R, Fristoe M, & Woodcock R (1974). *Goldman-Fristoe-Woodcock auditory skills test battery.* Circle Pines, Minnesota: American Guidance Service

Goldstein R (1967). Hearing disorders in children. Paper presented at the University of Oklahoma Symposium

Gray D, & Yaffe S (1983). Prenatal drugs. In C. Brown (Ed.), *Childhood learning disabilities and prenatal risk.* New Jersey: Johnson & Johnson Baby Products Company Pediatric Round Table, *9,* 44–49

Hall J (1964). Cochlea and the cochlear nuclei in asphyxia. *Acta Otolaryngologica,* Suppl. *194,* 68

Hammill D, Leigh J, McNutt G, & Larsen S (1981). A new definition of learning disabilities. *Learning Disability Quarterly, 4,* 336–341

Hardy W (1961). Auditory deficits of the kernicterus child. In C Swinyard (Ed.), *Kernicterus and its importance in cerebral palsy.* Springfield, IL: Charles C. Thomas, 255–266

Hasbrouck J (1980). Performance of students with auditory figure-ground disorders under conditions of unilateral and bilateral ear occlusion. *Journal of Learning Disabilities, 13,* 548–551

Hasbrouck J (1981). Prospects and procedures for the remediation of auditory processing disorders: a multi-discipline approach. Denver: Cherry Creek Schools

Hayes D, & Jerger J (1979). Aging and the use of hearing aids. *Scandinavian Audiology, 8,* 33–40

Heasley B (1974). *Auditory perceptual disorders and remediation.* Springfield, IL: Charles C. Thomas

Herr S (1969). *Perceptual communication skills.* Los Angeles: Instructional Materials and Equipment Distributors

Hind S, Goldberg J, Greenwood D, & Rose J (1963). Some discharge characteristics of single neurons in the inferior colliculus of the cat. II. Timing of the discharges and observations on binaural stimulation. *Journal of Neurophysiology, 26,* 321–341

Hirsh I (1967). Information input channels for speech and language: the significance of serial order of stimuli. In C Millikan and F Darley (Eds.), *Brain mechanisms underlying speech and language.* New York: Grune & Stratton, 21–38

Hurley R (1980). Speech protocols in the central auditory nervous system evaluation. In R Rupp & K Stockdell (Eds.), *Speech protocols in audiology.* New York: Grune & Stratton, 163–201

Hynd G (1981). Training the school psychologist in neuropsychology: perspectives, issues, and models. In G Hynd & J Obrzut (Eds.), *Neuropsychological assessment and the school-age child.* New York: Grune & Stratton, 379–404

Hynd G, & Obrzut J (Eds.) (1981). *Neuropsychological assessment and the school-age child.* New York: Grune & Stratton

Ivey R (1969). Tests of CNS function. Unpublished master's thesis, Colorado State University, Fort Collins, Colorado

Jerger J (1960). Audiological manifestations of lesions in the auditory nervous system. *Laryngoscope, 70,* 417–425

Jerger J (1964) Auditory tests for disorders of the central auditory mechanism. In W Fields & B Alford (Eds.), *Neurological aspects of auditory and vestibular disorders.* Springfield, IL: Charles C. Thomas, 77–93

Jerger J (1973). *Modern developments in audiology* (ed 2). New York: Academic Press

Jerger J (1975). Diagnostic use of impedance measures. In J Jerger (Ed.), *Handbook of clinical impedance audiometry.* Dobbs Ferry, New York: American Electromedics Corp., 149–174

Jerger S (1981). Evaluation of central auditory function in children. In R Keith (Ed.), *Central auditory and language disorders in children.* Houston: College-Hill Press, 30–60

Jerger J, & Jerger S (1971). Diagnostic significance of PB word functions. *Archives of Otolaryngology, 93,* 573–580

Jerger J, & Jerger S (1974). Auditory findings in brainstem disorders. *Archives of Otolaryngology, 99,* 342–350

Jerger J, & Jerger S (1975a). Clinical validity of central auditory tests. *Scandinavian Audiology, 4,* 147–163

Jerger J, & Jerger S (1975b). Extra- and intra-axial brainstem auditory disorders. *Audiology, 14,* 93–117

Johnson D, Enfield M, & Sherman R (1981). The use of the staggered spondaic word and the competing environmental sounds test in the evaluation of central auditory function of learning disabled children. *Ear and Hearing, 2,* 70–77

Jorgensen F (1980). *The complete handbook of magnetic recording* (ed 4). Blue Ridge Summit, PA: TAB Books, Inc.

Katz J (1962). The use of staggered spondaic words for assessing the integrity of the central auditory nervous system. *Journal of Auditory Research, 2,* 327-337

Katz J (1968). The SSW test—an interim report. *Journal of Speech and Hearing Disorders, 33,* 132–146

Katz J (1978a). Clinical use of central auditory tests. In J Katz (Ed.), *Handbook of clinical audiology* (ed 2). Baltimore: Williams & Wilkins, 233–243

Katz J (1978b). The effects of conductive hearing loss on auditory function. *ASHA,* 879–886

Katz J, & Burge C (1971). Auditory perception training for children with learning disabilities. *Menorah Medical Journal, 2,* 18–29

Katz J, & Harmon C (1981). Phonemic synthesis: testing and training. In R. Keith

(Ed.), *Central auditory and language disorders in children*. Houston: College-Hill Press, 145–159

Katz J, & Pack G (1975). New developments of differential diagnosis using the SW test. In N Sullivan (Ed.), *Central auditory processing disorders*. Omaha: University of Nebraska, 85–107

Keith R (1981). Summary of question and answer period. In R Keith (Ed.), *Central auditory and language disorders in children*. Houston: College-Hill Press, 175–184

Kiang N (1975). Stimulus representation in the discharge patterns of auditory neurons. In E Eagles (Ed.), *The nervous system*, Vol. 3. Human communication and its disorders. New York: Raven Press, 81–96

Kimura D (1961). Some effects of temporal lobe damage on auditory perception. *Canadian Journal of Psychology, 15*, 156–165

Kinsbourne M (1978). *Asymmetrical function of the brain*. Cambridge: Cambridge University Press

Kirk S, McCarthy J, & Kirk W (1968). *Illinois test of psycholinguistic abilities*. Urbana: University of Illinois Press

Konkle D, & Bess F (1974). A study of time-compressed speech with an elderly population. Paper presented at the American Speech and Hearing Association Convention, Las Vegas

Kurdziel S, Noffsinger D, & Olsen W (1976) Performance by cortical-lesion patients on 40% and 60% time-compressed materials. *Journal of the American Audiology Society, 2*, 3–7

Kurdziel S, Rintelmann W, & Beasley D (1975). Performance of noise induced hearing impaired listeners on time-compressed CNC monosyllables. *Journal of the American Audiology Society, 1*, 54–60

Lamarche S, & Rudmin F (1982). On CAP testing. *Hearing Aid Journal, 35(6)*, 46

Lasky E, & Cox L (1983). Auditory processing and language interaction. In E Lasky & J Katz (Eds.), *Central auditory processing disorders*. Baltimore: University Park Press, 243–268

Lasky E, & Katz J (Eds.) (1983). *Central auditory processing disorders*. Baltimore: University Park Press

Lehmann D, Creswell W, & Huffman W (1965). An investigation of the effects of various noise levels as measured by psychological performance and energy expenditure. *The Journal of School Health, 34*, 212–214

Levy F (1981). Central auditory testing in learning-disabled children. Master's dissertation, University of Witwatersrand, Johannesburg, South Africa

Liberman A, Cooper F, Shankweiler D, & Studdert-Kennedy M (1967). Perception of the speech code. *Psychological Review, 74*, 431–461

Lindamood C, & Lindamood P (1969). *Auditory discrimination in depth*. Boston: Teaching Resources Corporation

Lindamood C, & Lindamood P (1971). *LAC test examiners manual*. Boston: Teaching Resources Corporation

Linden A (1964). Distorted speech and binaural speech resyntheses tests. *Acta Otolaryngoligica, 55*, 32–48

Lindsay P, & Norman D (1972). *Human information processing*. New York: Academic Press

Loomis A, Harver P, & Hobart G (1938). Distribution of disturbance patterns in the human electroencephalogram, with special reference to sleep. *Journal of Neurophysiology, 1,* 413–430

Ludlow C (1980). Impaired language development: hypotheses for research. *Bulletin of the Orton Society, 130,* 153–169

Lynn G, Benitz J, Eisenbrey A, Gilroy J, & Wilner H (1972). Neuro-audiological correlates in cerebral hemisphere lesions: temporal and parietal lobe. *Audiology, 11,* 115–134

Lynn G, & Gilroy J (1972). Neuro-audiological abnormalities in patients with temporal lobe tumors. *Journal of Neurological Science, 17,* 167–184

Lynn G, & Gilroy J (1975). Effects of brain lesions on the perception of monotic and dichotic speech stimuli. Proceedings of: Symposium on Central Auditory Processing Disorders, University of Nebraska Medical Center, Omaha

Lynn G, & Gilroy J (1976). Central aspects of audition. In J Northern (Ed.), *Hearing disorders.* Boston: Little, Brown and Co., 102–118

Lynn, G, & Gilroy J (1977). Evaluation of central auditory dysfunction in patients with neurological disorders. In R Keith (Ed.), *Central auditory dysfunction.* New York: Grune & Stratton, 177–221

Magoun H (1963). *The waking brain* (ed 2). Springfield, IL.: Charles C. Thomas

Maki J, Beasley D, & Orchik D (1973). Children's perception of time-compressed speech using two measures of speech discrimination. Paper presented at the American Speech and Hearing Association Convention, Detroit

Manly W (1979). Phase, time, ears, and tape. *Audio,* April 52–68

Mattes J (1983). The Feingold diet: a current reappraisal. *Journal of Learning Disabilities, 16(6),* 319–323

Matzker J (1959). Two new methods for the assessment of central auditory functions in cases of brain disease. *Annals of Otology, Rhinology, & Laryngology, 68,* 1185–1197

McCandless G (1979). Impedance measures. In W Rintelmann (Ed.), *Hearing assessment.* Baltimore: University Park Press, 281–320

McCarthy J, & McCarthy F (1969). *Learning disabilities.* Boston: Allyn & Bacon

McCroskey R & Kasten R (1980). Assessment of central auditory processing. In R Rupp & K Stockdell (Eds.), *Speech protocols in audiology.* New York: Grune & Stratton, 339–389

McEwen B (1983). Hormones and the brain. In C Brown (Ed.), *Childhood learning disabilities and prenatal risk.* New Jersey: Johnson & Johnson Baby Products Company Pediatric Round Table, 9, 11–17

McNeil R & Prescott T (1978) *Revised token test.* Baltimore: University Park Press

McSpaden J (1982). Central deafness: Myth and manifestation. *Audecibel,* Fall, 16–19

Meyer M (1975). Paper presented at symposium on central auditory processing disorders in children with learning disabilities, Colorado State University

Mills J (1975). Noise and children: a review of literature. *Journal of Acoustical Society of America, 58,* 767–779

Milner B (1962). Laterality effects in audition. In V Mountcastle (Ed.), *Interhemispheric relations and cerebral dominance.* Baltimore: Johns Hopkins Press, 177–195

Miltenberger G, Caruso V, Correia M, & Love T, & Winkelman P (1979). Utilization of a central auditory processing test battery in diagnosing decompression sickness. *Journal of Speech and Hearing Disorders, 44*, 110–120

Morales-Garcia C, & Poole J (1972). Masked speech audiometry in central deafness. *Acta Otolaryngologica, 74* 307–316

Morest D (1964). The neuronal architecture of the medial geniculate body of the cat. *Journal of Anatomy, 98*, 611–630

Morest D (1975). Structural organization of the auditory pathways. In E Eagles (Ed.), *The nervous system*, Vol. 3. *Human communication and its disorders*. New York: Raven Press, 19–29

Moruzzi G, & Magoun H (1949). Brainstem reticular formation and activation of the EEG. *Electroencephalography and Clinical Neurophysiology Journal, 1*, 455–473

Moser H (1983). Genetics. In C Brown (Ed.), *Childhood learning disabilities and prenatal risk*. New Jersey, Johnson & Johnson Baby Products Company Pediatric Round Table, 9, 5–10

Musiek F (1983). Assessment of central auditory dysfunction: the dichotic digit test revisited. *Ear and Hearing, 4*, 79–83

Musiek F, & Geurkink N (1980). Auditory perceptual problems in children: considerations for the otolaryngologist and audiologist. *Laryngoscope, 90*, 962–971

Musiek F, & Geurkink N, & Keitel S (1982). Test battery assessment of auditory perceptual dysfunction in children. *Laryngoscope, 92*, 251–257

Musiek F, Pinheiro M, & Wilson D (1980). Auditory pattern perception in split brain patients. *Archives of Otolaryngology, 106*, 610–612

Musiek F, Wilson D, & Reeves A (1981). Staged commissurotomy and central auditory function. *Archives of Otolaryngology, 107*, 233–236

Myklebust H (1954). *Auditory disorders in children*. New York: Grune & Stratton

Myrick D (1982). A normative study to assess performance of a group of children aged 7–11 on the staggered spondaic word (SSW) test. In D Arnst & J Katz (Eds.)., *Central auditory assessment: the SSW test*. San Diego: College-Hill Press, 313–314

National Institute of Neurological and Communicative Disorders and Stroke (1981). News and comments. *Archives of Otolaryngology, 107*, 198

Nauta W, & Feirtag M (1979). The organization of the brain. *Scientific American, 241*, 88–111

Needleman H (1983). Environmental pollutants. In C Brown (Ed.), *Childhood learning disabilities and prenatal risk*. New Jersey: Johnson & Johnson Baby Products Company Pediatric Round Table, 9, 38–43

Netter F (1962a). *Otologic diagnosis and treatment of deafness* D Meyers, W Schlosser, & A Winchester (Eds.). Summit, NJ: CIBA Pharmaceutical Company

Netter F (1962b). *Nervous system*. Summit, NJ: CIBA Pharmaceutical Company

Noffsinger D, & Kurdziel S (1979) Assessment of central auditory lesions. In W Rintelmann (Ed.), *Hearing assessment*. Baltimore: University Park Press, 351–377

Noffsinger D, Olsen W, Carhart R, Hart C, & Sahgal V (1972). Auditory and vestibular aberrations in multiple sclerosis. *Acta Otolaryngologica Supplement, 303*

Oakland T, & Williams F (1971). *Auditory perception.* Seattle: Special Child Publications, Inc.

Olsen W, Noffsinger D, & Carhart R (1976). Masking level differences in clinical populations. *Audiology, 15,* 287–301

Olsen W, Noffsinger D, & Kurdziel S (1975). Speech discrimination in quiet and in white noise by patients with peripheral and central lesions. *Acta Otolaryngologica, 80,* 375–382

Orchik D, & Oelschlaeger M (1974). Time-compressed speech discrimination in children and its relationship to articulation. Paper presented at the American Speech and Hearing Association Convention, Las Vegas

Pinheiro M (1977a). Auditory pattern perception in patients with left and right hemisphere lesions. *Ohio Journal of Speech and Hearing, 12,* 9–20

Pinheiro M (1977b). Tests of central auditory function in children with learning disabilities. In R Keith (Ed.), *Central auditory dysfunction.* New York: Grune & Stratton, 223–256

Pinheiro M (1978). A central auditory test profile of learning disabled children with dyslexia. In L Bradford (Ed.), *Communication disorders: An audio journal for continuing education.* New York: Grune & Stratton 3(6)

Pisoni D, & Sawusch J (1975). Some stages of processing in speech perception. In A. Cohen & S. Nooteboom (Eds.). *Structure and process in speech perception.* New York: Springer-Verlag, 16–35

Protti E (1983). Brainstem auditory pathways and auditory processing disorders. In E Lasky and J Katz (Eds.). *Central auditory processing disorders.* Baltimore: University Park Press, 117–139

Public Law 94-142, 94th Congress (December 29, 1977), Section 121a5.

Rampp D (1980). *Auditory processing and learning disabilities.* Omaha, Nebraska: Cliff Notes, Inc.

Rasmussen A (194u). Studies of the VIII cranial nerve of man. *Laryngoscope, 50,* 67–83

Rasmussen A (1943). *Outlines of neuro-anatomy.* Dubuque, Iowa: W. C. Brown

Rasmussen G (1946). The olivary peduncle and other fiber projections of the superior olivary complex. *Journal of Comparative Neurology, 84,* 141–220

Rasmussen G (1960). Efferent fibers of the cochlear nerve and cochlear nucleus. In G Rasmussen & W Windle (Eds.). *Neural mechanisms of the auditory and vestibular systems.* Springfield, IL: Charles C. Thomas, 105–115

Reagan C (1973). *Handbook of auditory perceptual training.* Springfield, IL: Charles C. Thomas

Reagan C & Cunningham S (1976). *Differentiation of auditory perceptual skills.* Tucson: Communication Skill Builders, Inc.

Rees N (1973). Auditory processing factors in language disorders: The view from Procrustes' bed. *Journal of Speech and Hearing Disorders, 38,* 304–315

Reichman J, & Healey W (1983). Learning disabilities and conductive hearing loss involving otitis media. *Journal of Learning Disabilities, 16(5),* 272–278

Reite M, Zimmerman J, & Zimmerman J (1981). Magnetic auditory evoked fields: Inter-hemispheric asymmetry. *Electro-encephalography and Clinical Neurophysiology, 51,* 383–392

Report of the panel on communicative disorders (1979). National Advisory Neurological and Communicative Disorders and Stroke Council, U.S. Department of Health, Education, and Welfare

Rimland B, & Larson G (1983). Hair mineral analysis and behavior: An analysis of 51 studies. *Journal of Learning Disabilities, 16(5),* 279–285

Roberson H (1982). Tape recorder maintenance. *Audio, 66(4),* 33–37

Rose J, Greenwood D, Goldberg J, & Hind J (1963). Some discharge characteristics of single neurons in the inferior colliculus of the cat. I. Tonotopical organization, relation of spike counts to tone intensity, and firing patterns of single elements. *Journal of Neurophysiology, 26,* 294–320

Rose J, Gross N, Geisler C, & Hind J (1966). Some neural mechanisms in the inferior colliculus of the cat which may be relevant to localization of a sound source. *Journal of Neurophysiology, 29,* 288–314

Rose J, & Woolsey C (1949). The relations of thalamic connections, cellular structure, and evokable electrical activity in the auditory region of the cat. *Journal of Comparative Neurology, 91,* 441–466

Schain R (1977). *Neurology of childhood learning disorders* (ed 2). Baltimore: Williams & Wilkins

Schnitker M (1972). *The teacher's guide to the brain and learning.* San Rafael, CA: Academic Therapy Publications

Schoenfeld S (1975). The SSW test with children. Presented at expanded SSW workshop, Menorah Medical Center, Kansas City, Missouri, July

Schubert G, Meyer R, & Schmidt J (1973). Evaluation of the noise subtest of the Goldman-Fristoe-Woodcock test of auditory discrimination. *Journal of Auditory Research, 13,* 42–44

Selz M (1981). Halstead-Reitan neuropsychological test batteries for children. In G Hynd & J Obrzut (Eds.), *Neuropsychological assessment and the school-age child.* New York: Grune & Stratton, 195–235

Semel E (1976). *Semel auditory processing program.* Chicago: Follett Publishing Company

Sever J (1983). Maternal infections. In C Brown (Ed.), *Childhood learning disabilities and prenatal risk.* New Jersey: Johnson and Johnson Baby Products Company Pediatric Round Table, 9, 31–38

Shepard L, & Smith M (1981). Evaluation of the identification of perceptual-communicative disorders. Laboratory of Educational Research, Department of Education, University of Colorado

Shimizu H, Brown F, Capute A, & Mahoney W (1981). Auditory brainstem response in children with minimal brain dysfunction. Paper presented at the American Speech and Hearing Association Convention, Los Angeles

Shirinian M, & Arnst D (1982). Patterns of the performance-intensity functions for phonetically-balanced word lists and synthetic sentences in aged listeners. *Archives of Otolaryngology, 108,* 15–20

Simopoulos A (1983). Nutrition. *Childhood learning disabilities and prenatal risk.* In C Brown (Ed.). New Jersey: Johnson and Johnson Baby Products Company, Pediatric Round Table, 9, 26–31

Sinha S (1959). The role of the temporal lobe in hearing. Master's thesis, McGill University

Slavin S (1978). Information processing defects in delinquents. In L Hippchen (Ed.). *Ecologic-biochemical approaches to treatment of delinquents and criminals.* New York: Van Nostrand Reinhold Co., 75–104

Sloan C (1980). Auditory processing disorders and language development. In P Levinson & C Sloan (Eds.), *Auditory processing and language: Clinical and research perspectives.* New York: Grune & Stratton, 117–133

Smith B, & Resnick D (1972). An auditory test for assessing brainstem integrity: Preliminary report. *Laryngoscope, 82,* 414–424

Smock S (1982). Central auditory skills in juvenile delinquents. Master's thesis, Colorado State University

Sohmer H, & Student Q (1978). Auditory nerve and brainstem evoked responses in normal, autistic, minimally brain damaged and psychomotor retarded children. *Electroencephalography and Clinical Neurophysiology, 44,* 380–388

Speaks C (1975). Dichotic listening: A clinical or research tool? Proceeding of a symposium on central auditory processing disorders, Omaha: University of Nebraska Medical Center, 1–25

Sprague R, & Sleator E (1976). Drugs and dosages: Implications for learning disabilities. In R Knights & D Bakker (Eds.), *The neuropsychology of learning disorders.* Baltimore: University Park Press, 351–366

Springer S, & Deutsch G (1981). *Left brain, right brain.* San Francisco: W H Freeman and Company

Stander H (1945). *Textbook of obstetrics.* New York: Appleton-Century-Crofts

Stark R, & Tallal P (1979). Analysis of stop consonant production errors in developmentally dysphasic children. *Journal of Acoustical Society of America, 66,* 1703–1712

Stark R, & Tallal P (1981). Perceptual and motor deficits in language-impaired children. In R Keith (Ed.), *Central auditory and language disorders in children.* Houston: College-Hill Press, 121–144

Stevens K, & House A (1972). Speech perception. In J Tobias (Ed.), *Foundations of modern auditory theory,* Vol. 2. New York: Academic Press, 1–62

Stillman R (1980). Auditory brain mechanisms. In P Levinson & Sloan (Eds.), *Auditory processing and language: Clinical and research perspectives.* New York: Grune & Stratton, 1–18

Strauss A, & Lehtinen L (1947). *Psychopathology and education of the brain-injured child.* New York: Grune & Stratton

Streissguth A (1983). Smoking and drinking. In C Brown (Ed.), *Childhood learning disabilities and prenatal risk.* New Jersey: Johnson and Johnson Baby Products Company Pediatric Round Table, 9, 49–56

Studdert-Kennedy M (1974). The perception of speech. In T Sebeok (Ed.), *Current trends in linguistics,* Vol. 12. The Hague: Mouton, 2349–2385

Sweetow R, & Reddell R (1978). The use of masking level differences in the identification of children with perceptual problems. *Journal of the American Auditory Society, 4,* 52–56

Sweitzer R (1977). Team evaluation of auditory perceptually-handicapped children. In R Keith (Ed.), *Central auditory dysfunction.* New York: Grune & Stratton, 341–360

Swoboda P, Morse P, & Leavitt L (1976). Continuous vowel discrimination in normal and at risk infants. *Child Development, 47,* 459–465

Tallal P, & Newcombe F (1978). Impairment of auditory perception and language comprehension in dysphasia. *Brain and Language, 5,* 13–24

Tallal P, & Piercy M (1974). Developmental aphasia: Rate of auditory processing and selective impairment of consonant perception. *Neuropsychologia, 12,* 83–93

Tallal P, Stark R, Kallman C, & Mellits D (1980). Perceptual constancy for phonemic categories: A developmental study with normal and language impaired children. *Applied Psycholinguistics, 1,* 49–64

Thal D (1978). Examination of information obtained from tone tests and its relationship to the language skills of children with developmental dysphasia. Doctoral dissertation, the City University of New York

Thal D, & Barone P (1983). Auditory processing and language impairment in children: Stimulus considerations for intervention. *Journal of Speech and Hearing Disorders, 48,* 18–24

Thurlow M, & Ysseldyke J (1979). Current assessment and decision-making practices in model LD programs. *Learning Disability Quarterly, 2,* 15–24

Toman P (1969). Oral language of the disabled child. *Journal of Learning Disabilities, 6,* 38–41

Trehub S (1976). The discrimination of foreign speech contrasts by infants and adults. *Child Development, 47,* 466–472

University of Nebraska Medical Center (1975). *Proceedings of a symposium on central auditory processing disorders.* Omaha

Ventry I (1980). Effects of conductive hearing loss: Fact or fiction. *Journal of Speech and Hearing Disorders, 45(2),* 143–156

Weber H (1977). The selection of hearing aids. Unpublished paper, 1–12

Webster D (1983). Effects of peripheral hearing losses on the auditory brainstem. In E Lasky & J Katz (Eds.), *Central auditory processing disorders.* Baltimore: University Park Press, 185–199

Weener P (1974). Toward a developmental model of auditory processes. *Acta Symbolica, 5,* 85–104

Wepman J (1958). *Auditory discrimination test.* Chicago: Language Research Associates

White E (1977). Children's performance on the SSW test and Willeford battery: Interim clinical report. In R Keith (Ed.), *Central auditory dysfunction.* New York: Grune & Stratton, 319–340

Whitfield I (1967). *The auditory pathway.* Baltimore: Williams & Wilkins

Wiederholt J (1978). Adolescents with learning disabilities: The problem in perspective. In L Mann, L Goodman, & J Wiederholt (Eds.), *Teaching the learning-disabled adolescent.* Boston: Houghton-Mifflin Company, 9–27

Wiig E, & Semel E (1976). *Language disabilities in children and adolescents.* Columbus, Ohio: Charles E. Merrill

Willeford J (1976). Central auditory function in children with learning disabilities. *Audiology and Hearing Education, 2(2),* 12–20

Willeford J (1977a). Differential diagnosis of central auditory dysfunction. In

L Bradford (Ed.), *Audiology: An audio journal for continuing education.* New York: Grune & Stratton, 2(4)

Willeford J (1977b). Assessing central auditory behavior in children: A test battery approach. In R Keith (Ed.), *Central auditory dysfunction.* New York: Grune & Stratton, 43–72

Willeford J (1978a). Sentence tests of central auditory function. In J Katz (Ed.), *Handbook of clinical audiology* (ed 2). Baltimore: Williams & Wilkins, 252–261

Willeford J (1978b). Expanded central auditory test battery norms. Unpublished

Willeford J (1980a). Central auditory behaviors in learning disabled children. *Seminars in Speech Language and Hearing, 1,* 127–140

Willeford J (1980b). Central auditory processing questionnaire: an unpublished survey of central auditory services in ASHA accredited programs

Willeford J, & Billger J (1978). Auditory perception in children with learning disabilities. In J Katz (Ed.), *Handbook of clinical audiology* (ed 2). Baltimore: Williams & Wilkins, 410–425

Willeford J, & Mealler J (1979). Evaluation of the Lindamood auditory conceptualization test as an auditory test. Unpublished study, Colorado State University

Willette R, Jackson B, & Peckins I (1970). *Auditory Perception Training (APT).* Chicago: Developmental Learning Materials

Windle W (1950). *Asphyxia neonatorum.* Springfield, IL: Charles C. Thomas

Witelson S (1977). Early hemispheric specialization and interhemisphere plasticity: An empirical and theoretical review. In S Segalowitz & F Gruber (Eds.), *Language development and neurological theory.* New York: Academic Press, 213–287

Witkin R (1971). Auditory perception—Implications for language development. *Language Speech and Hearing Services in the Schools,* Monograph 4, Washington, D.C.: American Speech and Hearing Association, circa 1971, 31–52

Wood N (1972). Auditory closure and auditory discrimination in young children. *Proceedings of the first annual Memphis State symposium on auditory processing and learning disabilities,* 136–152

Woodcock R (1976). *Goldman-Fristoe-Woodcock auditory skills test battery technical manual.* Circle Pines, Minn.: American Guidance Service, Inc.

Woolard H, & Harpman J (1940). The connexions of the inferior colliculus and of the dorsal nucleus of the lateral lemniscus. *Journal of Anatomy, 74,* 441–458

Worthington D (1981). ABR in special populations. Paper presented at ABR Workshop, Cleveland, Ohio

Worthington D, Beauchaine K, Peters J, & Reiland J (1981). Abnormal ABR's in children with severe speech/language delays. Paper presented at the American Speech, Language and Hearing Association Convention, Los Angeles

Yost W, & Nielsen D (1977). *Fundamentals of hearing.* New York: Holt, Rinehart, & Winston

Young M (1983). Neuroscience, pragmatic competence, and auditory processing. In E Lasky & J Katz (Eds.), *Central auditory processing disorders.* Baltimore: University Park Press, 141–161

Young M, & Protti E (1981). Central auditory perceptual testing: Implications regarding children's hearing aid fittings. *Hearing Aid Journal, 34,* 8–42

Zemlin W (1968). *Speech and hearing science: Anatomy and physiology.* Englewood Cliffs, NJ: Prentice-Hall

Zwislocki J (1975). The role of the external and middle ears in sound transmission. In E Eagles (Ed.), *The nervous system*, Vol. 3. Human communication and its disorders. New York: Raven Press, 3, 45–55

Author Index

Subject Index